WHEN
SOMEONE
YOU LOVE
HAS
CANCER

WHEN SOMEONE YOU LOVE HAS CANCER

Dana Rae Pomeroy

IBS PRESS, INC.
SANTA MONICA, CALIFORNIA

Cover & book design by Melvin L. Harris & Susan C. Muller-Harris
Computer Graphics by Melvin L. Harris
Type Composition by Susan C. Muller-Harris
Editing by BettyClare Moffatt

IBS PRESS, INC.
744 Pier Avenue
Santa Monica, CA 90405
(213)450-6485

IBS PRESS FIRST PRINTING, JULY, 1991

Library of Congress Cataloging-in-Publication Data
Pomeroy, Dana Rae, 1946--
    When someone you love has cancer / by Dana Rae Pomeroy
        p.   cm.
    Includes bibliographical references.
    ISBN 1-877880-06-X
    1. Cancer--Patients--Family relationships. 2. Cancer--Patients--
Home care. 3. Terminal care. 4. Adjustment (Psychology)
I. Title.
RC262.P64   1991
649.8--dc20   91-482
                                                                  CIP

ISBN 1-877880-06-X

Made in the United States of America

Dedication

This book is dedicated to each of you who must deal with the reality of cancer in your family, to the hospice nurses everywhere who make living with cancer a possibility, and to my late husband, Walter F. Sinner and my dad, Oren D. Pomeroy, Jr.

Acknowledgements

This book would not have been possible without the support and assistance of a number of people, spread across the United States. Among the special people who helped in the creation of this book:

Shelly Webb, who allowed inclusion of examples of the battle she and her husband, David Tomkins, fought with cancer.

Judy Elsen, our hospice nurse in Juneau, Alaska, who encouraged me in the beginning and provided moral support and technical assistance with the final draft.

The Friday Writers, who poked, prodded, edited, encouraged and demanded the very best.

Dr. Josefina Magno for her review and encouragement and for writing the forward to this book.

And especially my husband, Al Link, who has supported and encouraged me every step of the way since the first day he learned of my dream for this project.

Contents

Foreword

Taking care of a loved one with a terminal illness is never easy. The primary caregiver, usually the spouse, is burdened with many responsibilities in addition to the tremendous emotional stress that accompanies the struggle with cancer.

When Someone You Love Has Cancer caught my attention because it was written by the wife of a man who was dying of lung cancer at a time in their relatively young lives when, for the first time, things had begun to work out for both of them—financially, professionally and emotionally. It is therefore a story that is something that we might watch on our television screens, except that this story is real life. It depicts the pain, the fears, the worries, the anger, the guilt, the grief, the confusion and every human emotion that accompanies a diagnosis of cancer.

It is a blessing that Dana Rae Pomeroy had the insights and the gift of writing, because these enabled her to make a journal of everything that happened to herself and to her husband in the course of her husband's illness. She describes the emotions that accompanied each visit to the doctor's office and each stay in the hospital, as well as the day to day struggle as she tried to care for him in their home. But the more important part of the book is the fact that she faithfully describes all the practical things that she had to do in order to cope with each painful and frustrating moment, and to help her husband deal with all of them in his own way.

When Someone You Love Has Cancer provides the guidance and the practical suggestions that anyone struggling with a diagnosis of cancer, whether as a patient or as a family member, will find very useful. It is written in simple language; it is well organized; it has samples of important documents such as living wills, record keeping, etc. It even has chapters on how to deal with the grief that follows the death of the loved one.

The rare thing about this book is the fact that it was written out of the personal experiences of someone who lived through the ordeal in our present day and age. It was not researched out of textbooks or scientific publications and then compiled into a "how to" manual. Reading the book is like reading someone's personal diary and one can identify with and relate to the many situations that are described in it.

I feel that *When Someone You Love Has Cancer* will be an important source of help for patients and families who find themselves in this difficult and trying time in their lives.

JOSEFINA B. MAGNO, M.D.
PRESIDENT
INTERNATIONAL HOSPICE INSTITUTE

Introduction

NOVEMBER 7TH -
I begin to fear the chemo isn't working. It's 2:00
a.m. and I feel so lost and alone...

When this book was conceived, I was nursing my husband, Walt, through his brief battle with lung cancer. I was generally frightened, sometimes angry, often confused and doing things I had never dreamed myself capable of handling.

And I was searching for additional guidance, someone or something to help me understand what I was feeling, help me more easily accomplish all that needed to be done and maybe tell me what else I could do. While there were any number of books by doctors, psychologist, nurses and ministers, nowhere could I find a basic "How to Get Through This" book with practical advice and some degree of empathy. Nor could I find a non-clinical book by someonewho had been through this and truly knew something about my feelings, my concerns, my confusion.

This book is not technical, clinical or medical. It is intended to be practical and helpful. It was written to answer some of the many questions that occur during the course of a terminal illness, in this case, cancer.

I do not set myself up to be an expert; rather, I hope to be a friend. I have viewed this book as a series of conversations I wish I could have with you when you need understanding, answers or a broad shoulder. How much easier it would be if you could just pick up the phone and call me. Since you can't, and since I want to be there for you, I've tried to write this book as if you had called or come by the house and asked questions, like the ones I asked while we were coping with my husband's cancer, like the questions others have asked me since then.

I was more fortunate than most. My good friend Shelly and her husband Dave had been battling lymphatic cancer for the three years of their marriage. They provided both practical and emotional support. There are numerous references and experiences in this book provided by Shelly when she learned of the project. She deserves a very special "Thank You" from all of us for her sharing and her caring.

A big part of the drive behind this book has been the knowledge of how much easier it was having Shelly's support, recognizing that a situation such as we had is in many ways unusual. Throughout this book, I want each of you to know that you are not alone; others have been there and others are there for you. Hopefully I can provide answers to some of the questions and doubts you are experiencing and help you better understand and cope with the battle you are facing.

In spite of loving and supportive friends and family, a wonderful doctor and a terrific hospice team, there were so many times I felt so helpless, like I was groping in the dark. I was also, at times, just plain frustrated. I vowed that whatever our outcome, I would sit down and do whatever I could to make the fight easier for anyone else facing the same battle. This book is the fulfillment of that promise to myself.

This book is divided into sections, many of which are further divided into specific questions and concerns. The Contents will help you find my thoughts about and experience with a specific issue. If you want to read the book from front to back, fine. If you're looking for answers to a specific situation, go directly to that section. I suggest you turn first to the checklist in Appendix A for the immediate basics.

This book has been written for the primary caregiver, spouse, parent, child or best friend of the cancer patient. It may also be helpful for all family members and close friends who will be involved with you and the patient. You may wish to read parts of it to your patient or suggest they read the book on their own. It may help them understand what you are going through and help them realize that you are at least aware of what they may be feeling and facing. It may also make it easier for them to see your concerns for what they really are; practical considerations in your loved one's best interest. I have included excerpts from my personal journal, entries made during the months of Walt's illness, throughout the book. I hope these private reflections may help you to accept yourself as human and realize that you truly are not alone in your concerns, fears, resentments and day-to-day battles with guilt and despair.

DANA RAE POMEROY
APRIL, 1991

1

Accepting the Diagnosis

-SEPTEMBER 4TH -

Results from Friday's tests show cancer cells and tumor cells. the doctor gave us the news at noon. There is no way to describe the feeling one has at this time. Walt wanted some time alone, so I went to Mom's, called Deb to come out and fell apart. We will, of course go South for a second opinion and treatment.

I know of nothing to compare with the overall feeling of hearing the words, "It's cancer." The physical and emotional reactions are subconscious and overwhelming. "Why?" is one of the first major reactions. We received Walt's diagnosis after a year of upheavals, priority shifts and a wonderful summer. It was a time, in fact, when everything seemed to be coming together. The three and a half years we had been married had been a continuous series of ups and downs—financial crises, housing concerns, various problems with his children—but we were now on our way. We had spent every possible moment that summer on the new boat Walt had been wanting since he'd moved to Alaska seven years earlier. I was thirty-nine years old and had just started my own business; Walt was forty-seven, had a job he thoroughly enjoyed and lived life to the fullest. We had money in the bank, were anticipating income from the settlement of my grandfather's estate and were planning to finish the last half of our partially completed home.

Why did this happen to us? Why now? Quite honestly, I still have no answers. Technically this happened because of Walt's exposure to asbestos while in the military service. Why now? Technically because asbestos cancer requires ten to fifteen years to manifest the tumor.

Technical answers were not, of course, what I was looking for. I had gone through the same questions in 1978 when my father died of cancer. There were no answers then, either. Walt and Daddy were much alike and their responses were similar.

Walt said, "The Man Upstairs wrote the day of my birth, the way of my life and the date of my death before he sent me down here." Although they were both willing to accept this as fact, they both fought every minute of every day against their illness.

I honestly believe there are no answers to my questions, just as there are probably none to similar questions you are asking. At least not at the time they're asked, and maybe never. I can remember the day we received Walt's diagnosis. I drove to my mother's house, called my sister and sat in a chair, crying and repeating, "Why, Why, Why?" There were no answers then and none now.

The important thing is to quit asking "Why?" and start asking "How?" How do we treat it? How do we beat it? How do we make Walt more comfortable? How do we reach the required calorie level? How do we use the available medications? How do we pay the bills? How do we live with it?

You can learn to live and cope with cancer. It will take lots of time, lots of energy and lots of help from family, friends, agencies and organizations. It will also take lots of patience and probably a lot of tears. But it can be done.

Whether you have just received such a diagnosis or you are well into your battle with cancer, please go to Appendix A and read the First Week Check List before continuing with this book.

2
Emotions Throughout

-November 4th -

It's 2:00 a.m. and Walt has been up and down like a yo-yo since going to bed at 6:30. ...He ate very little today and lost it all at 8:30. ...He's been so groggy, Judy suggested we stop the Percocet. I'm on a real downer tonight, tired and frustrated and out of patience.

It's okay to be angry. In the beginning, when you receive the diagnosis, and anytime thereafter. This situation isn't fair and it isn't easy. Although it may be character-building it certainly isn't anybody's idea of fun.

Bear in mind that anger takes many forms, his, hers, and yours. And you are sometimes going to bear the brunt of it. Because you're angry and frustrated and feel so helpless you may both lash out. He or she may yell at you when in reality he's yelling at the cancer, the frustration, the feeling of helplessness, the fear.

If we're honest, this is probably the most frightening issue any of us have ever faced. Anger is a very real way of coping with fear. This is probably the single most important thing our friend, David, taught me in our phone conversations the week before he died of lymphatic cancer. David and Shelly's experiences are included throughout this book.

The cancer patient may seem to frequently "pick" at you: "You smoke too much"; "All that coffee isn't good for you"; "You need more sleep"; and on and on. They aren't really picking at you, however. Instead, they're concerned for you and your well being and they're often afraid that you aren't taking care of yourself because you're caring for them. They also feel helpless to do anything about their concern. Bear this in mind while you grit your teeth and count to eighty-seven!

You too will feel anger. I openly warned friends right up front that there would likely be times when I was short, hostile, snappy or just plain disagreeable and I apologized in advance. I was all those things at one time or another. Fortunately, they were very understanding.

While your loved one may well take his or her anger out on you at times, you certainly cannot be angry with one you love when they are so sick, right? Not true!

Although you are not dealing with the physical aspects of cancer yourself, you are experiencing all the emotional aspects. Quite often your feelings of helplessness are more intense than the patient's.

In addition, you are probably dealing with insurance forms, bills, increased expenses and decreased income, all on a minimum of sleep. This does not make for an even temper.

How about the day when you finally hit the end of your rope and yell back at your loved one? Well, you feel guilty, but only briefly, I hope. After all, didn't you hit levels of impatience when he or she was well and things looked great? There should be no more guilt now than there was then! Don't set yourself up to be Super Person. That's setting yourself up for guaranteed failure.

I'll probably never forget the night I really blew up at Walt. I was tired and behind on paperwork and generally feeling out of control. My sister Debby came over to move several boxes from our den to her new apartment. Normally, Walt would have hauled the boxes out while Deb and I gossiped over coffee, but he was too weak for lifting and was tied to the oxygen condenser in the interest of breathing. At the moment, I didn't think about how frustrating that must have been.

He began insisting that Deb shouldn't be carrying the boxes, that we should call one of the guys to help and on and on it went, him protesting from his seat at the kitchen table, me retorting from the kitchen, Deb caught in the middle, staring into a cup of coffee.

Finally I slammed a rice container down on the counter and pointed out that she and I had probably moved more boxes more often than any five men over the past ten years. I then stalked out of the room. Deb left a few minutes later without the boxes.

I was consumed with guilt and also in tears. How could I have possibly shouted at Walt when he was so sick? What kind of a jerk was I?

Then the phone rang. It was Deb, "Sorry I left so suddenly, but I was going to explode if I didn't laugh!"

"Laugh!" I choked through tears. "Sorry, I can't find the humor."

"Well, you missed the punch line. As soon as you left the room, Walt glared at your back and muttered 'I hope she broke her damn Tupperware!' Honestly, you two are like a couple of three year olds sometimes."

Grinning by now, I returned to the kitchen and Walt. "Tupperware has a lifetime guarantee, remember?" I teased.

I apologized, he apologized, we hugged, and life went on. But the memory of that event helped me maintain perspective when tempers got short, nerves were raw and guilt about feeling anger tried to take over.

Anxiety

Anxiety is different from anger. Anger is generally directed at a specific person, thing or situation. Anxiety is apprehension. We usually can't define a specific danger or threat, but we have an overall feeling that is undirected toward a specific cause.

Anxiety is common for anyone contemplating the possibility of his own death or the death of a loved one. Difficult as it may seem, the best way to deal with anxiety is to break it down and define its causes. By attempting to identify the individual reasons for your feelings of anxiety, each fear, each concern can be dealt with individually. Think of it as making swiss cheese out of a big yellow brick. A solid wall is overwhelming, but a wall full of holes can be overcome. Your anxiety, or your loved one's anxiety, is a wall. By looking for the causes of the anxiety, you can remove bricks from the wall, eliminating one more barrier of emotional upheaval. Your loved one's inability or unwillingness to discuss causes of anxiety can result in not only emotional swings, but restless nights. If you feel unexpressed anxiety is creating further problems for your loved one, talk with your doctor or hospice nurse. There are medications that help reduce the physical effects of repressed anxiety.

Denial

Denial is often the only method people can use, initially, to cope with the trauma and the fears that are an integral part of the cancer diagnosis. Walt never denied that he had cancer. But he steadfastly denied that he might die, until ten hours before his death. That denial was critical to his well being during the times when he chafed at the restrictions resulting from his growing weakness and his dependency on the oxygen condenser and oxygen tanks. Meantime, until his last two weeks, I also denied the possibility of Walt's death on a conscious level. In looking back, I think there were, in reality, many times my subconscious explored the possibility of his death.

Denial is not the same thing as hope or faith. The dictionary defines these words for us as follows:

FAITH: unquestioning belief; complete trust or
     reliance.
HOPE: a feeling that what is wanted will happen.
DENIAL: a refusal to believe or accept.

Faith and hope were the two things that kept me going through Walt's illness.

Denial creates some very real problems. The first major issue, especially if you have made no preparation for the eventuality of death, is that in the event the cancer patient does not win the battle, the surviving spouse is left with very real problems. Practical considerations, such as Power of Attorney and Wills, are addressed later in the appendix. How these are dealt with is entirely dependent upon the individual personalities involved.

The second problem with denial is that there are so many little ends left loose and you don't know how to tie them up. Thankfully, Walt and I had talked about death in the abstract on two or three occasions, when acquaintances had passed away, and I knew how he felt about artificial life support, cremation, sad and mournful memorial services. Equally fortunate, we knew each other's likes and dislikes in almost all areas of life, so there were not so many questions as there could have been.

Denial can also create feelings of isolation. If either of you is denying the fact of the illness, the other one feels isolated with their concerns and fears. If this is the case, find someone, anyone to talk with: a friend, pastor, counselor, American Cancer Society volunteer. Look for support groups in your area. If you can't talk with your spouse, because he or she is denying the illness, find a support person or support group for yourself. If you are the one denying the illness, help your spouse find someone they can talk with about their feelings.

Denial comes and goes without being verbalized. Walt and I took a trip down the Oregon coast, because we recognized he might never see it again nor have the opportunity to show me something that was so important to him. We applied for Social Security disability to help pay the bills while he recuperated. I had him sign a power of attorney to prevent problems with his insurance company and the bank, should he not make it. We paid a thousand dollars for a double recliner to watch football games together. It was a perpetual see-saw over the brief ten week period after the diagnosis.

In David and Shelly's case, it was a little different. David knew he had been beating the odds against death for several years. Although he never quit fighting, never quit believing he could win, he did make preparations for the eventuality of death and worked to help Shelly prepare for that time.

They had planned and saved for a future together, yet Dave was adamant about taking care of the "just in case" plans. These plans included "just in case" something were to happen to either one of them. Their wills and living wills were prepared and kept current. They discussed and wrote into their wills what each wanted or did not want in the way of burial and funeral arrangements. When David retired from the U.S. Army Reserves, they discussed and decided on the best plan to use in collecting his retirement benefits. Titles to vehicles and all financial accounts, as well as the house, were joint with right of survivorship. Both were involved in their financial planning and they discussed everything There were no secrets about how much money they had, what insurance policies existed and where everything was.

Even with this practical approach, Shelly and David practiced their share of mutual denial. They spent a lot of time planning for when "Dave is back on his feet", "Next year we will..." Yet this did not stop their planning for the other possibility.

If denial is the patient's primary method of coping with cancer, there is little you can do to change the fact. Don't try. You are doing them no favors in forcing them to face negative possibilities which they are not ready to cope with. This is equally true for you although, quite frankly, at some point you will probably be forced to give up the denial method of coping.

I witnessed this two years ago with another good friend. John had been given no hope and a prognosis of ten months. He had accepted the diagnosis and the prognosis and had immediately begun dealing with all the practical arrangements for everything from potential extended home care to a current will, trust funds and even the funeral services.

While Sue intellectually accepted the facts and his preparations, she totally denied the fact that he was dying throughout almost the entire process. Not only was this emotionally crippling for her, it made coping more difficult for John and helping more difficult for her hospice and her friends.

Denial comes and goes. Denial is not necessarily bad, but it will not work as a singular, long-term coping method.

Fear

The dictionary defines fear as "alarm... apprehension... concern". I felt all of these things during our bout with cancer. Something which can't be anticipated, predicted or controlled promotes various levels of fear within each of us. We all want the familiarity of the known and predictable. Instead we are suddenly dealing with what seems to be a world of unknowns, over which we have little or no control.

Your loved one may be dealing with their own set of fears: What if people ignore and avoid me? What if I'm all alone and nobody cares? What if I become totally dependent upon my spouse, child, or friends? What if I become ugly or disfigured? What if I'm no longer loveable?

All of these fears may be part of your loved one's emotions during the course of the illness. Our society has placed such an unreasonable (in my opinion) emphasis on appearance and ability, that loss of one's normal appearance and independence is a staggering blow to many individuals. Do all that you can to be sure your loved one knows that you do love them, that these physical changes make no difference in your feelings or attitude towards them as the person you care about.

You will probably have your own set of fears. What is going to happen next? Can I truly care for the most important person in my world? What will I do if I have to go on without them?

Recognize and admit to these fears. They are very real and very normal and hiding them or hiding from them isn't going to help. Some of these fears are part of the grieving process necessary for dealing with a critical illness.

I was particularly vulnerable to fear when we were facing a crisis or late at night when I was alone. Talking with Shelly, a member of my family or the hospice nurses helped tremendously. If it was late and no one was available, I talked to God and wrote in my journal.

Don't be ashamed of having these fears. The one thing I was unable to do was discuss with Walt his fears and mine. As he continued to deny the possibility of anything but full recovery to me, he couldn't admit to these fears. After he died, however, the hospital Chaplain and Pastor George both told me that Walt had discussed his fears with them and there had been several lengthy discussions about life after death. Walt felt sure that if he did die, we would meet in the future.

Grief

Grief is a perfectly normal reaction to be experienced and dealt with at this point. Shelly and I experienced periods of grief throughout our husbands' illnesses: grief at the time of diagnosis, grief over the pain and discomfort being experienced, grief for each time some treatment didn't work as expected and grief over the possibility of losing our husbands. This grief is normal and healthy as long as it is recognized and allowed. It is an inherent part of coping with cancer for both you and your loved one. Tears are healthy and healing.

Take time to do your own grieving. Get in touch with and admit to your emotions. It is only natural to feel grief at the fact that your loved one is experiencing pain and fear and frustration. You may feel grief over happier moments lost to the illness. Quite possibly you feel grief at the possibility of losing your loved one. Ignoring these feelings and denying yourself the right to grieve is one more building block in the wall of stress.

Guilt

Guilt is normal, but not healthy. In all honesty, I could have driven myself over the edge with guilt. Why didn't I insist Walt see a doctor last spring, when he mentioned being tired all the time? Why didn't I agree to his taking another two weeks without pay in June, to spend more time on the boat? Why hadn't I worked harder to get my business going? Why hadn't I tried to strengthen our relationship with his daughters? Why had I spent so much time at my computer evenings or reading late at night? During his illness, how could I have gotten so impatient when he had me up every hour to check on medications? And on and on and on.

But wait. I'm me and he loved me because I'm me. We truly had and did all the things that were really important to us. That's what counts.

Guilt can make you crazy, but you can't go back at this point and rewrite the story. You can do everything possible to make this period positive and satisfying. You can recognize that you are the person your loved one loves and cares for. He or she has probably suspected, on rare occasions, that you may not be perfect!

Everyone is aware of the need to be understanding, tolerant and accepting of the patient. Apply the same principle to yourself. Don't feel guilty about needing this same consideration. Be aware of your own fright, anger, frustration and hurt. Be understanding with yourself as well.

Whatever you and your family feel is okay. Whatever the patient feels is okay. You do not have to do anything about the patient's feelings except listen to them. You do not need to understand them or to change them. You are not personally responsible for the disease nor its ramifications. Regardless of your reactions and feelings, you have nothing to be truly guilty about.

It is essential that family members attend to their own needs, while allowing the patient responsibility for their own health. It is imperative that spouses, family members and friends encourage patients to do what they can for themselves and give them love, support and affection when they demonstrate independence. To expect that family members can meet all the patient's emotional needs, and still pay attention to their own, is unreasonable at best.

Resentment

Here is another demon emotion that is probably going to rear its head. Resentment is often a part of anger. And acknowledging this emotion can put you back into the vicious cycle of guilt.

There is no reason why you and your loved one shouldn't feel resentment. After all, resentment is bitterness or hurt, brought on by a person or action. Admit that you may be bitter about the diagnosis, the prognosis, the demands the illness is placing on both of you. Few of us can not be hurt by unthinking words or actions that may occur as a result of stress, frustration or just plain being tired.

Your loved one may resent you or other family members for his or her feelings of helplessness and dependency. He or she may resent your constant encouragement to eat more or other actions they see as nagging. They may well resent the possibility that they will not be here to see future events and you will be.

You, on the other hand, may periodically resent your loss of freedom to come and go, as well as the budget constraints brought on by the illness. You may resent the fact that your loved one seems to ignore all your efforts to provide attractive and appealing meals. You may resent your loved one's dependence upon you, particularly if they have been the strong one in the past. And you may resent the fact that there is a possibility that he or she is going to die and leave you here alone to cope with the world.

You may not, quite frankly, be able to talk with one another about your feelings of resentment. I encourage you to find someone to talk to, even if it's the dog. Even if it means "talking" to a piece of paper with a pen. Denying resentment can create a festering wound of anger and frustration. Resentment is normal but like guilt, unhealthy if it is ignored or denied.

This is not the time of your life to rebuild your entire personality so you can do and be all the things you should. In fact, right now "should" and "ought" do not apply to your behavior. The only time these two words must be considered a part of your vocabulary is when they apply to diet or treatment requirements that may not appeal to either of you, but are necessary for recovery. Right now you simply need to be the person you are and be there for the cancer patient in the same way you always have been. Whenever people started sentences with "You should" or "You ought to", I usually tuned them out. There is no way someone who hasn't been there and isn't you has a clue to what you are feeling and what you are coping with.

3

Attitude

-OCTOBER 29 -

It is all so frustrating. I try to be positive, but right now it's late and I'm tired and Walt's had a rotten day, which means so have I.

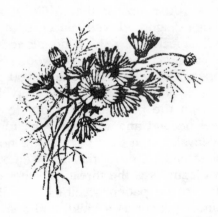

A ttitude is unique to each individual, their personalities and their relationships.

Hugh Prather says in his book *Notes to Myself,* "I can change my response to a feeling, but I can no more get rid of it than I can get rid of myself. When I disown a feeling I do not destroy it, I only forfeit my capacity to act it out as I wish." Attitude is unique to each individual, their personalities and their relationships. One of the first things I hope you realize is that while your loved one may have been diagnosed with cancer, both of you must deal the with cancer. He or she is not alone in their fears, anxiety and concerns and neither are you.

Be as open with your loved one as you possibly can. If something is bothering you, speak up. If you need something from the patient, ask. Your loved one still needs to feel needed and worthy. Don't turn them into more of an invalid than they already are nor treat them like a helpless child. One of the major emotional effects of a cancer diagnosis is the threat, whether conscious or unconscious, to the patient's self-esteem. People often treat the cancer patient as a child, and sometimes not a very bright one! Remember, this is still the loving adult you care for and admire.

Encourage your loved one to do what they can. David folded laundry, paid the bills, made salad for dinners, etc. Shelly purchased a handcart to allow him to continue taking the garbage cans to the curb. Just because one has cancer doesn't mean they are suddenly incapable or incompetent to handle day to day living.

It is very important to allow the individual their dignity. Your loved one is the same person they have always been, with the same feelings, needs and priorities. At this point, a problem has cropped up and some adjustments may need to be made for current levels of ability.

Even though Walt was often weak or easily tired, he wanted to spend time with his new niece and nephew. The twins had been born the day before Walt went in for the initial tests. Using the portable oxygen tank, with a spare in the trunk, we would visit my sister. Walt might nap in their recliner for part of the visit. But when he wasn't napping, he was a pro at calming one or both of the four week old twins, freeing my sister and I to do some of the many duties required by two brand new babies.

You and Your Loved One

Please do all you can to maintain open and honest communication between yourself and your loved one. You both need to openly discuss your fears and hopes, your concerns and love for each other and for yourselves. During the first weeks following the diagnosis of cancer, it is important to establish a basis for this type of communication. The patient needs to be allowed and encouraged to express his or her feelings and concerns.

Determine the basis for your relationship. The attitudes, feelings and moods you possessed before the diagnosis are the basic attitudes, feelings and moods you will have after the initial shock wears off. There are no magic changes. Don't treat your loved one any differently than you did before they were ill. They probably do not need or want special treatment. The recognition that there are no automatic changes in attitude as a result of terminal illness is not restricted to you and your loved one. It extends to parents, children, sisters and brothers. If there has been conflict, lack of attention or veiled hostility in the past, it will not magically go away.

Methods of coping with cancer are unique and individual. Walt's attitude was not the same as mine. Walt's attitude was not the same as Dave's. In some respects, Shelly's attitude and mine also differed.

Dave wanted to know the details of available options and treatments and he and Shelly were able to spend long hours discussing the pros and cons and what was to happen if the treatments didn't work. In our case, I wanted all the information I could get and was willing to face the odds which we were dealing with. In fact it was necessary for me to know all I could. Yet Walt and I never talked about what to do if he lost the battle. We spent our time encouraging each other and talking about what we would do when he recovered. Although I knew our odds were slim, and had talked at length to the doctors about what to expect and how to deal with his discomfort and pain, Walt never took a look at the possibility he wouldn't make it until the night he died.

Friends and Relatives

Your attitudes toward the illness and its effects will, to a large degree, dictate the overall attitudes, actions and reactions of friends and family. The critical issue here is their acceptance of the fact and their acceptance of the patient. I remembered what my father went through during his illness. Co-workers and acquaintances didn't drop by because they didn't know what to say or how to act or they couldn't cope with terminal illness. The loneliness resulting from their attitude was harder for my father than many other conditions of his illness. I vowed we would not go through the same thing.

We were honest with our close friends. We said Walt had cancer, there would be some rough times and we needed to see our friends often. I told them the diagnosis. When we returned from extensive testing and initial treatment in Seattle, I shared the prognosis with them. I also talked with them about what I expected, what I anticipated and about Walt's feelings. We were fortunate in having many friends who came to visit both at home and in the hospital. In a couple of instances, I advised visitors about what was and was not acceptable as a topic of conversation as I knew some individuals had a tendency to bring up and discuss unsettling or upsetting situations. As a result, our friends accepted the facts, knew they could talk openly with us, ask questions and offer the types of assistance and support we needed. Because I was open about our hopes and fears, they could accept Walt's frustration and my periodic need for a strong shoulder and a good cry.

Knowing we would talk openly about the situation if they wanted to, knowing we would welcome visitors, knowing that Walt might or might not be awake, knowing that his physical, mental and emotional state could change literally from day to day or hour to hour, they also knew we both loved and needed them. There was very little hesitancy on their part.

We had some of our best weekends with friends after Walt's return from Seattle. He had been puttering all spring and summer with a workshop addition to the house. After our return from Seattle, several couples came over on three successive Saturdays. The guys brought their tools and finished the wall supports, stuffed insulation and hung sheet rock. The women brought needlework and knitting. At the end of the day I served a big lasagna dinner or had a fish fry. They didn't ask if there was "anything they could do". They simply called and said "Here's what we're going to do this weekend."

Walt was involved with the work, even though he could physically do nothing during the last two work parties. We moved a comfortable chair into the shop area and he supervised, answering questions about his preferences. He enjoyed having our friends at the house and they felt that they were, finally, doing something for us as their feelings of helplessness and frustration were often as great as ours.

Dave and Shelly were equally open. When they got tired of seeing the four walls of their home and needed a change of scenery and people, Shelly would simply let family and friends know they were ready for a night out. Many times, they would go over to dinner and find their hosts had "reserved" a couch for Dave so he could lay down. Friends were understanding if they had to leave early because Dave was having difficulty balancing the pain medication. Other times, friends dropped by for a quick cup of coffee, bringing special deserts for Dave. They were aware of his high calorie diet and went out of their way to provide tasty, tempting treats for him.

Your Children's Friends and Associates

Where there are youngsters at home, it is equally important to contact the adults they come in frequent contact with and advise them of the situation. Your children will probably go through many of the emotions described in this book. If their teachers, scout or brownie leaders and the parents of their playmates know that the children are facing upheavals and changes at home, they will be better able to understand and deal with changes in the child's actions, behavior and emotions.

What Happens to Sex?

Sex is rarely discussed and often ignored in discussions of cancer. It is a critical area to those of us facing the terminal illness of a spouse. The fact that your loved one has cancer does not change the fact that they are still a complete person and the person you love. Sex can become a very touchy area if you are not open with each other.

Walt and I were best friends and able to talk about almost anything. To be very candid, after we got Walt's diagnosis, during those times that he was feeling fairly good, we had some of our most tender moments. Maybe it was because we were able at that point to fully appreciate the moment and the emotions involved. It also brought us so close in every way. It may be up to you to initiate any discussion or any action toward sexual intimacy. Many times a cancer patient feels that the cancer somehow makes them unlovable from a physical standpoint.

Some people are still harboring the feeling that cancer is contagious. Some patients feel that you can't possibly love someone who is sick. Remember that one of cancer's major side effects is its attack on the patient's self esteem.

From your point of view, you may be afraid the victim isn't feeling good enough to engage in any sexual activity. You may fear he or she will think you are being selfish for wanting something so down-to-earth when they are dealing with a critical illness. Don't make assumptions.. Talk about sex, if it's comfortable for you.

If it isn't, initiate lovemaking as you have in the past, making it clear that it is the loved one's decision to accept or not.

Sex is not just the act of making love, but more importantly, the simple touching, hugging and loving gestures that reassure your spouse that he or she is still loved, cared for and needed as an entire person. During the final days, Walt and I would sit with our arms around each other and talk and laugh about special times in the past. The sharing and caring seemed to fill that part of our relationship.

Sex is a very personal and individual issue, determined by the two people involved. I can only encourage you to deal with sex much as you have always done. When your wife had a blinding headache or your husband had a pulled muscle, physical sex was replaced by loving tenderness. However, when one of you had a perfectly awful day and simply needed reassurance, you probably provided that reassurance with tangled sheets and a short night. The situation here is the same: treat the pain, respect any discomfort and then love each other's strain and stress away.

4
Taking Care of Yourself

-NOVEMBER 6TH -

I hated having to tell him he had to stay at the hospital, he wanted to come home so badly. It's so frustrating, but I haven't had more than three hours of sleep at a time in the last four days. It's probably a good idea for the two of us to get a couple of day's and night's rest. He needs to be more comfortable physically before he comes home again.

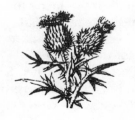

Y our mental and physical health is just as important as the patient's. I ignored mine. Had Walt's illness been an extended one, I would have been in a great deal of trouble.

Shelly dealt with Dave's illness for three years. She forced herself to eat properly, exercise regularly and get away from the house periodically. She took classes one night a week to provide necessary mental challenge and new ideas and concepts.

Again, this is a unique area, based on personalities and the course the cancer is taking. I cannot tell you what is right for you, what you ought to do or should do. Right or wrong has no bearing on your comfort level or your emotional well being.

Most people think of the many things that have to be done to care for the patient, yet little thought is given to the caregiver. It is just as important to take care of yourself as it is to care for the patient.

It's easy to neglect yourself when facing a medical crisis with a loved one. It's easy to say "He is more important right now, I'll take care of myself later, when he's back on the mend."

You cannot care for someone else if you are drained from stress and exhaustion or have developed health or emotional problems yourself. If you take care of yourself, you will be physically and emotionally able to care for your loved one when you are needed most.

Plan your self care with the long term in mind. Shelly visualized herself preparing for a marathon. She knew she needed to be in good physical and mental health to be able to care for David when the going got rougher than it already was. Consequently, she made it a point to be physically, mentally and emotionally in good health. This included exercise and continuing with her outside interests, such as art classes and reading.

There will be times when, just like your loved one, you will either not feel like eating at all or you'll want to eat everything in sight! We all deal with stress in different ways. My mother eats; I have a tendency to lose my appetite; my brother escapes into sleep with early to bed, late to rise and naps in between. For the majority of us, stress affects our eating habits.

Since you are probably dealing with nutrition for your loved one already, extend that concern to yourself. Do the best you can to prepare balanced meals and to get the proper nutrition when you're eating out. You may want to check with your doctor and see about vitamins that provide the extras needed when stress is draining the body of normal nutrients.

Physical exercise helps you both physically and emotionally. It does not have to be a formal visit to your local spa or health club, but could simply be thirty minute walks daily. Incorporate exercise into your daily life. Park your car five blocks from the hospital and walk to and from it. Use the stairs instead of the elevator. Walk around the grounds or the parking lot if your loved one is napping or having x-rays or tests. Try isometric or gentle stretching exercises when you're housebound.

A visit to a health club or spa may be the "escape" that you need. If this is the case, set up a regular schedule and make it a part of your life.

Shelly spent hours cutting and stacking firewood for the winter. That was something that she and David used to do together and the familiar outdoor activity gave her the outlet she needed to exercise, think and have some time alone.

Do not feel guilty because you want and need an afternoon off to do something for yourself. Make arrangements to have someone else stay with your loved one so you can have lunch with a friend, pursue a hobby, take the dog for a walk. That time is vital to you and to your loved one. Remember your loved one needs the time away from you just as much as you need the break.

About two weeks after Walt had come home with the oxygen condenser, a friend called and said he wanted to come spend some time with Walt. If I needed some time out, he'd be there for two or three hours. I made a luncheon date with three friends. After having my hair cut and styled, I met them for a luxury lunch downtown. I arrived home after a two hour mini-vacation feeling one hundred percent better than when I had left. Walt was in better spirits because he felt I had been given a treat. The outing had a positive effect on my feelings about myself, my outlook, my temper and my patience. You're working hard to help your spouse be comfortable and cared for. You deserve a bonus now and then.

Someone once said that life is easier than you think. All you have to do is accept the impossible, do without the indispensable, and bear the intolerable. Attempting to accomplish this is a very real part of living with cancer. The fear of the unknown, dealing with the results of treatments, the pain, the anger, the frustration are all contributors. The constant exposure to your loved one's pain or discomfort creates a stress level of its own kind. All this is added to the myriad details involved with the paperwork for insurance claims and the constant outgo of dollars.

Then there are the outside forces over which you have no control. These include the pressure of meeting appointments with doctors, specialists, laboratories; the necessity of working with other people's schedules; the possiblity of long hours of nursing, combined with longer hours of paperwork.

Internally, there may be the often justified feeling that people are expecting more from you than you can give. You may feel that you have to be a Super Caregiver, the best in the world. You may also be uncomfortable asking for help or accepting help when it's offered.

Hopefully you can locate an associate, friend, or organization that will help you talk it out. Hospice and home health care agencies usually have counselors who are trained to assist you and your loved one in dealing with the various emotions of cancer.

Often you don't need anyone to give advice as much as you need someone to listen and simply be there. For me that "listener" was sometimes my journal. Writing down my concerns, my frustrations, my feelings was a healthy outlet for me. Sometimes writing them down helped me let go of them somewhat. Sometimes as I wrote, an alternative or an answer would come to me. Many times I wrote out my anger on a piece of paper, then tore up that piece of paper as if I were destroying the actual anger or frustration. Whatever works for you is okay.

Give yourself permission to relax. Recognize that you cannot be all things to all people and learn to accept help when it's offered. This was one of the hardest things for me to learn to do gracefully and gratefully. Normally a logical person, I felt that I had to do it all myself.

You might look around for stress management courses. Check with your local hospice group. Even if you don't require their medical or volunteer assistance, you may benefit from their informal support groups made up of others in the same situation. If possible, talk to people who have gone through what you are experiencing now. These people are often the greatest resource available for practical tips and support. Check to see if the "I Can Cope" program offered by the American Cancer Society or a program similar to it is available in your area.

Now is the time to get your annual physical. Discuss the stress that you are under with your physician. You do not want or need your body to fail when you are needed to be at your best.

Taking care of yourself is not a selfish activity. Wanting and needing time for yourself, time to do things that are important to you, is not something to feel guilty about. When you take the time to ensure your health, you are doing this for your loved one. You will be able, physically and emotionally, to support them through their battle. You will be stronger and able to handle whatever the outcome. You will be ready to provide the strong support required if the going gets rough.

Decide what is right for you and your loved one. Don't let other people tell you how they think you should or should not handle a situation. People often make statements about how they feel something should or should not be handled. You may feel guilty about doing it differently. Yet you know your situation better than anyone else. It's fine to ask for ideas but make your own decisions. Don't let anyone push you into doing something that you are not comfortable with. You and only you are the one that has to live with it.

Hugh Prather said in *Notes to Myself,* "...Forgive yourself daily—hourly if need be—for punishing yourself for being human."

Guilt is the way we punish ourselves for not being perfect. Try to follow Prather's advice. Tape a copy of this reminder to the bathroom mirror or the kitchen refrigerator. Its message is as true for the cancer patient as it is for you, the caregiver.

"I wish it were over" is not something to be guilty about. It is another way of saying "I wish we were not feeling this pain and this frustration." It is a feeling of love and compassion for both yourself and your loved one,. You are the two most important people in the world in this situation.

5
Do It Now

SEPTEMBER 25TH -

It's beautiful here. Walt was a genius to suggest the coast trip. Our campsite is grassy and wooded, we walked along the water's edge at the beach and explored the wreck of the Peter Iredale, before returning to the motor home for dinner.

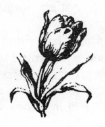

If there are things you've talked about doing, things you've wanted to do, DO IT NOW! This is important to both you and the patient. Quite frankly, the only restriction on your activities is your loved one's physical abilities and their feelings about being able. Maybe you've been promising yourselves a gourmet dinner at that new exclusive restaurant. Do it now. Maybe it's something as simple as planning a drive out through the State Park, but housework and chores always made you put it off until next weekend. Do it now. Maybe you've always talked about a trip to the Virgin Islands. If your spouse is up to it, do it now. I am not advocating total irresponsibility, but I do not encourage total practicality at this time either.

Fortunately Walt and I had done many of the things we wanted to do, when we wanted to do them. Since my father's death in 1978, my family was not so prone to put all of our plans into the future. Like most folks, however, there were a number of little things we had talked about doing and kept putting off.

The weekend before going to Seattle, Walt was released from the hospital in Juneau for four days. Sunday he was anxious to be outside, after all the hospital time. We piled into the car and drove out to EagleCrest and down to Fish Creek, both beautiful, natural areas that he wanted to absorb. Simple local drives we had previously put off in favor of chores at home, since we knew those spots would still be there when we got around to going.

With the expenses of a new boat and starting a new business, our budget rarely included going out to dinner. However, the night we got into Seattle, in spite of being horribly uncomfortable, Walt wanted to go out to dinner. He figured if he went into hospital he would get plenty of room service! We treated ourselves to a quiet and intimate dinner, in a delightful gourmet restaurant in our hotel, china, crystal, linen, the whole nine yards. It cost us well over one hundred dollars, unheard of for two practical folk like us, but it was worth every penny of it, given the events of the next ten days. When things got rough, we relived the feelings of elegance and luxury and reviewed the melt-in-your-mouth menu items, promising ourselves a repeat performance when he was released from treatment.

As Walt went through initial treatment and started feeling better, he began planning to show me the Oregon coast, something we had often talked of doing and had on our agenda for the following summer. He wanted to see it now. His doctor agreed we could go for a few days, as long as we checked in with him as soon as we returned.

Walt had lived for several years on the Oregon coast and loved the area; I had never been there. In spite of what was going on, in spite of questionable finances and an uncertain future, the trip was important to both of us. I made a number of phone calls and the day after Walt was released from Swedish Hospital, we picked up a twenty-four foot motor home and headed out of Seattle. I had never driven anything that big in my life, but I learned how quickly. Walt was weak and tired easily, but we had a beautiful trip from Newport Beach up to Astoria. We were able to have breakfast whenever we wanted; we could pull into a rest area or one of the small state parks whenever Walt got tired so he could nap for an hour; he could nap before dinner. I'm well aware that many people thought we were crazy and irresponsible, but it was a very special time for us and worth every penny I paid.

Shelly is also a strong proponent of the Do it Now and Ignore the Shoulds and Oughts Theory. Dave was in a lot of pain the summer before he died, in spite of all the pain medication he was taking. Yet he continued to want to do as much as possible. His day consisted of getting up, getting ready for work, lying down until she drove him to work, lying down at the office until it was time to begin work. His breaks and lunch hours were taken on the couch. Then home to lie down again until supper time. They spent months with this routine.

He wanted a chance to use their recently acquired, seventeen foot skiff and get out and camp, something they had done extensively the first two years of their marriage. They decided to take a camping trip to a small island not far from Juneau. Shelly spent the week preparing for the trip: gathering all the gear; buying a lawn lounge chair for Dave; making lists; preparing food. Packing included not only food, water, tent and standard camping supplies but also an arsenal of medications. She alerted several of us with larger boats and radios to their plans. We agreed to cruise by and check the camp throughout the two days. If Dave and Shelly got into trouble, help was nearby.

Saturday morning while Dave rested on the couch, Shelly loaded the camping gear and hitched up the boat trailer. Accompanied by their dogs, they headed to the marina, launched the skiff and took off for Shelter Island. They made it out to the island with no trouble. Shelly immediately set up Dave's spot, so he could lay down again, then went about setting up camp.

The weekend proved to be just what they needed. It was warm and sunny; Dave was able to rest comfortably and read while Shelly kept camp, played with the dogs and enjoyed some long overdue relaxation. They talked for hours. Friends came by to check on them and were waved on their way. This was a very special time alone for them.

Returning home turned out to be much more difficult. Strong winds had come up early in the morning, resulting in a heavy tide and three foot swells between the island and home. It was a real physical challenge for Dave and Shelly to get the boat off the beach and into the incoming tide and wind. Dave was exhausted by the time they got back to the mainland. But the island trip was well worth the exhaustion and the struggles.

That weekend became one of their favorite memories. They relived the weekend time and again when things got really rough. Any logical, rational person would have said they shouldn't have attempted the trip (and several did say so). These people were probably right. Emotionally, however, it was the right thing to do. It gave Dave and Shelly both a tremendous lift and made the following weeks and months easier to deal with.

Do what is right for you and your spouse. Don't listen to what others think you should or shouldn't do! Instead, follow your heart.

6

Friends and Relatives

-SEPTEMBER 12TH -

Tony showed up about 11:00 tonight, had received the message I left after the doctor's rather negative prognosis. He let me babble until 3:00 a.m. and mopped up a lot of tears in the process.

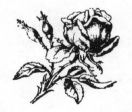

So many times we want to help and don't know what to do. This section suggests ways in which you can assist and things you can do to help the patient, the caregiver and the family.

The most important thing you can offer is yourself. Just knowing you are available and caring means a great deal to both the cancer patient and their loved ones.

There are three major DOs to keep in mind:

Be available
Be supportive
Be a willing and quiet listener.

There are three major DON'Ts:

Please don't wait to be asked.

For many of us, trying to adjust to the shock and cope with all the changes and new requirements in our lives is difficult at best. Asking for help is one more thing we must learn to do. Many times we don't know what to ask, who to ask, how to ask. There is a very human tendency not to impose our own problems and concerns on other people who are busy with their own lives.

Please don't tell the patient or caregiver what they should do or how they should feel.

Helpful suggestions of available alternatives are wonderful at a time like this, but no one can tell someone else how to cope with the possibility of death.

Please don't treat the patient like a child just because he or she is ill or try to make them feel any more of an invalid or patient than they already are.

Cancer is a major enemy of an individual's self esteem and feelings of self worth and it is important to allow the patient all the freedom, responsibility and capability they need and desire.

The helping examples provided below come from my own experience of what people did to make life more bearable; what I wish people had done, and what I have done in similar circumstances.

Visit

Visit frequently, even if only for a few minutes. New faces and fresh subjects are particularly welcome to the housebound or those in the hospital for any period of time.

Recognize there will be both up days and down days for the patient As a result, there will be ups and downs for the caregiver and family as well. Realize that their reactions on a down day have nothing to do with you personally.

Offer to keep the patient company while the spouse is out running errands. My husband hated the thought of a babysitter, but couldn't be left alone at the house. However he thoroughly enjoyed visits from the guys where he used to work. They made it a point to let me know when they were coming and how long they could stay so I could get out without Walt feeling he was being watched over or dependent. Bear in mind that being dependent is a very new and unnerving experience for most of us. Anything you can do to help without creating feelings of dependence is of major assistance.

Practical and Moral Support

Accept the patient's or caregiver's need to alternately discuss the illness and deny it; denial may be a major part of eventual acceptance. Conversely, denial may be the only way the individual can deal with the situation.

If travel is necessary for treatment, you can assist in making the travel arrangements, contacting support groups in the other city, finding a house-sitter or pet sitter if one is needed, applying for travel assistance if available from the local American Cancer Society or the insurance company. Coping with cancer means dealing with an incredible array of details and many people are not very good at this, particularly when most of their energies are directed toward the patient and their own emotions.

Ask if the patient or caregiver would like your moral support when they have a doctor's appointment or are scheduled for out-patient therapy of some type. This is particularly appreciated if the patient would otherwise have to go alone. It is also appreciated if the caregiver is going to be sitting in a hospital or clinic waiting room for an hour or so.

Sharing the diagnosis with others makes living with it easier for everyone in the long run. However, it isn't easy to make those calls. The family may appreciate offers to advise church groups or social or fraternal organizations or even other friends about the diagnosis. I had neither the time nor the inclination to make the dozens of calls necessary to advise and update all the people who knew and cared for Walt and myself. Friends and family made any number of calls for me. I learned later that without these calls many people would have been hurt because they didn't know of the diagnosis. Don't ask "Can or should I call anyone?" Instead you might ask "Would you like me to call the Elks? the American Legion? your church?"

If the family isn't aware of support groups, you can help by either giving them the phone numbers or offering to contact hospice, American Cancer Society, Public Health Nursing or others. There are a number of organizations available. But someone has to find the time to make all the calls needed.

Information may be the thing the family needs the most. You may know where the patient and family can go for various types of help. Or you may have the time and talent to find out.

Most of us are unaware of the many agencies and groups established to help us with this type of situation. You can help make the family aware of what's available. You can also be aware of the circumstances in which agencies are not able to offer assistance and thus save a lot of time with frustrating negative contacts.

At a very practical level, you can help the family with the paperwork necessary to obtain the help available. Social security and Veterans Administration, for example, require that reams of paperwork be completed to qualify for the disability benefits. In addition, they base waiting periods on the date of application instead of the date disability occurred. This is also true of some group disability insurance firms. You can collect the forms and establish the initial contact person. You can also assist in filling out the forms and returning the forms. All of this is of tremendous help.

If there is a large amount or variety of medication required, you can help make arrangements with the drugstore to either set up a charge account or accept standard charge cards so the billings can be paid monthly as the insurance checks arrive. This type of arrangement makes life so much easier, especially if someone else needs to pick up prescriptions or the patient is requiring new medications often.

If you're good at detail and organization, and if the family will accept that type of help, you can set up a system for tracking the medical bills. Perhaps you can set up the system outlined in this book. Terminal illness is a very expensive experience, but many things can be done to reduce the immediate fiscal pain at least.

If you have access to a copying machine, you can make copies of the insurance claims, Social Security forms and/or Veterans Administration forms. Having copies of any claims filed is of tremendous help yet can be a major hassle for the primary caregiver to accomplish.

Gifts, Treats and Necessities

Bring fresh flowers. Not necessarily expensive arrangements delivered by strangers, but a couple of carnations or a single rose delivered by you personally with a smile.

Provide books and magazines, those little extras you frequently pick up when out shopping. If you've noticed magazines around the house that are not subscription, pick up the latest issues. Ask if there are particular weekly or monthly magazines they read. How about a favorite author's new book?

Does the patient or caregiver need supplies to continue a project or hobby? My sister helped when she brought over the two skeins of yarn I needed to finish an afghan.

Call when leaving for the store and ask what the family needs from the grocery store.

Children

If there are children, you can arrange field trips, picnics, walks on the beach. You can help them with school work or attend one of their school functions. Mom or Dad would love to be able to do everything, but there are only twenty-four hours in any given day.

Perhaps someone is needed to watch the children while the parents see the doctor or go for out-patient treatment.

Food

Bring the family complete meals, ones that can be eaten immediately or refrigerated or frozen for later use. It is extremely frustrating to have someone deliver a meat loaf when you are out of potatoes or have no canned vegetables left.

The week before Sue's husband died I took over a goodie box. The spaghetti sauce was accompanied by spaghetti noodles and French bread rolls. The meat loaf was accompanied by vegetables and a box of mashed potato mix. The casserole meal included onion rolls to compliment the ingredients of the casserole. And there were all the makings of a salad bar packaged separately so that the salad wouldn't go bad after a couple of days. Sue commented that those were the only meals they ate. It seemed like everything else that came into the house required some grocery item they didn't have on the shelves.

Most cancer patients have extremely high calorie and protein requirements while fighting the tumor(s), so if you enjoy baking, your treats will be a welcome addition to efforts to tempt the appetite.

Bring an extra plate of goodies just for those folks who may stop by for coffee. When people brought over snacks for Walt, I felt they had to be reserved for him alone, whether he ate them or not. I actually felt guilty feeding them to other people who stopped by to visit. (Spouses and other caregivers do not always apply great logic in this situation.)

Asking Questions

Ask specific yes or no questions in order to help. The question "Do you need anything?" will generally get a "No" response. The question "I'm going by the store, do you need eggs or milk?" will probably elicit a positive response or a list of other required items.

"Could I pick the kids up for a day of fishing Saturday?" will probably get a more positive response than, "Is there anything I can do?"

One of the critical issues too often unrecognized by even caring friends and relatives, is that of taking care of the person who is taking care of the patient. I don't think this can be emphasized enough. I can almost guarantee the caregiving spouse or family member is not taking care of themselves most of the time.

The caregiver needs your help, support and understanding just as much as the patient does. They are facing many of the same fears and frustrations. They are often trying to play round-the-clock nurse at the same time that they are coping with the financial and practical issues of the current situation.

Take five minutes and think about being in this situation yourself. If you had the same concerns and responsibilities and couldn't leave your house for seven days, what would you want to have at the house? What would you want to do if you could leave the house for two hours at the end of that seven days? What would you miss most about not being able to run out whenever you wanted to? What would be the major drawback of being house-bound for one week? This will give you a general feeling as to what the patient needs.

Fortunately I didn't often have to ask for help. People just did what needed to be done.

If they were coming to the house they called and said, "We're headed for the grocery store, how's the dairy supply?" When Walt was in the hospital for several days they would kidnap me for an hour's change of scenery, a good hot meal and a shoulder to cry on. My brother-in-law would simply call the hospital and say, "Dinner will be on the table in thirty minutes and your niece and nephew need to hug you." It is unbelievable how much better life looks when these things occur.

7

Children and Cancer

I need to talk to the girls. Their mother said she'd told them Walt has cancer, but I feel like I need to reassure them. I remember how I felt when I found out about Daddy.

Y ears ago I read a statement regarding the obligation we have to our children. In essence it said
that it was our duty to prepare them to deal with
the world as it really is and not the world as we have
known it or as we want it to be. Walt's girls were going
to have to deal with a portion of the world I had known.
It was something I wished they didn't have to go through.
But their father's illness was the reality.

How and what do you tell children about the illness
and the potential problems ahead? While there are as
many different situations as there are human beings, my
overall feeling and the feelings of those I have talked
with, is that children have the right and the need to know
what is happening in their lives.

My first experience with cancer occurred when I was
five years old and my grandfather had leukemia. I don't
remember a great deal about the situation. One thing I do
remember is that the illness was never hidden from my
cousin and myself; we were assigned duties to help
Grandpa Ray. He had to use crutches to get around and
he always had an afternoon nap. One of my main memories is that my cousin and I were responsible for locating
his shoes (we each were assigned a foot, so to speak),
helping get them tied and then getting his crutches after

his afternoon nap. While I don't remember a great deal of detail, we were aware that Grandpa Ray was sick and that we all needed to help.

My next experience occurred when I was twelve years old and my best friend was diagnosed with leukemia. While I wasn't provided with great medical detail, Mom and Dad explained to me that Emily had an illness that had settled in her blood. They said she would be tired lots of the time and couldn't always attend school. Sometimes she would have to go to a special hospital where they would help make her feel better. The only caution was that because of the illness we had to be more careful when we played with her, because the slightest bump could cause a bruise.

There was no shielding me from the fact of the illness, no keeping me isolated from my friend, only the necessary cautions for her well being. As Emily's condition worsened, my folks explained to me that in spite of all the doctors were trying to do, Emily might not live to be my best friend forever. The facts were not presented in a negative manner, nor as a fatalistic philosophy, but merely pointed out so that I could help Emily and understand why some days I couldn't see her or some days she might be grouchy or in pain. The overall perception that I had was that the doctors were doing all they could, but perhaps God needed Emily in Heaven to help him more than we needed her down here to play with us.

When my father was diagnosed with cancer, I was an adult of thirty-two. Still I was the child of the man who was sick. My parents lived in Alaska and I lived in Minnesota. Mom didn't come right out and say it was cancer, only that there were some abnormal cells discovered when Dad had his hernia operation. Knowing their doctor's name, and suspecting that Mom was leaving out more than she was telling, I contacted the doctor in Alaska. He called it cancer. Within two weeks of knowing, I was on a plane to Alaska from my home in Minneapolis.

During my ten days there my parents were honest with the facts they had. This time was a little different for me. This was my father. And he and Mom were going through some of their own types of denial, hope and grief. Daddy looked and felt pretty good. We went fishing one day and hiking on another occasion. He moved a little slower but we were able to believe this was a problem that would go away. I returned to Minneapolis and made arrangements to move to Alaska permanently. I'd fallen in love with the place and looked forward to being close to my family again.

As time went on, it became clear that Dad was not getting better. My folks made arrangements to go to the Mayo Clinic and we met in Seattle, me on the way to Alaska, while they were on their way to Minnesota. When they came back home six weeks later it was obvious that we were dealing only with a matter of time. Daddy and I talked about his illness and the knowledge that everything that could be done wasn't enough. While one is never ready to accept the death of a loved one, the openness and love we shared before he died was possible only because there was honesty about the illness and prognosis. That openness made it much easier to cope with his death that Christmas.

Dealing with children of any age is an emotional trauma when terminal illness is involved. At a time when you are trying to cope with some very frightening news, you must also help your children try to understand what's happening. There is no right or wrong way to handle this phase of the situation. Shelly and David had no children. Walt had three teenagers from a previous marriage. Mr.

Kwan, a delightful gentleman introduced to me by our hospice nurses, had two children under the age of ten. In today's families, there are so many different situations and family structures and varying circumstances that I can only relate to you my experiences and those of Mr. Kwan, as well as the ramifications of our actions.

In our case, Walt had three daughters between fifteen and twenty-two, all living within ten miles. Two of the girls were out on their own; the youngest had spent the summer with us and then gone to live with her mother when Walt first got sick. Although the girls loved their father, theirs had never been a close family. Throughout our brief marriage, they lived sometimes with us, sometimes with their mother and her husband, sometimes in their own apartments.

As soon as we received the diagnosis, I called their mother and asked her to have all the girls at her house that evening. I wanted to talk with them about what was going on and what we would be doing as far as travel to Seattle, Walt's treatment, the future and so forth. I hoped to be able to give the girls what facts we had and talk about their questions and concerns. Remembering how my parents had dealt with the cancer issue and how much easier it was to accept the known rather than fear the unknown, Walt and I agreed this was the approach we wanted to take. While they would know their father was seriously ill, we felt they should also know what we were going to do to try and make him well. I was hoping to enlist their cooperation in frequent visits.

Walt's girls did not relate well to his illness nor to the possibility of death. I think a great deal of the problem was our inability to sit down and discuss the issue, since the unknown is always much more frightening than the known. Their visits to their father were few and far between, but they had been so when Walt was well and healthy, so this was no big change. On a couple of occasions, I did call the girls and tell them that if they wanted to see their father they should do so in the next day or so. The first time was a false alarm; the second time they waited too long.

Looking back, I have wondered if there were things that could have been done differently. However, each of us must deal with these situations as best we can when they occur.

The girls did come to the house together the day he died. I told them the positive details of his feelings, his being at home and being surrounded by friends at all times. We talked about his attitude throughout the illness and the positive feelings he expressed the last day, about a life well lived and friends made and love shared. He was ready to leave us when his time came. Their critical concern was that he was not alone when he died and on that point they were reassured.

My friend Sue faced a similar situation two years ago with her husband's grown children, all living out of town. The summer of his diagnosis, the kids all came for a weekend birthday celebration. Following that weekend, they called sporadically for "progress" reports. When John begin failing, Sue asked and then begged that they come see their father. Their responses ranged from comments that a four hour drive was much too exhausting to the statement that they couldn't afford a plane ticket and didn't want to take time off work. In reality, they simply weren't ready to face the fact that their father was becoming more seriously ill each week. They continued to deny to themselves the possibility of John's death. They never did make it back to see their father before he died.

Why do I present these negative examples? Because at least half of you are dealing with step children, shared custody, multiple families. Because these reactions, particularly from older or grown children, are not in the least uncommon. Because these types of reactions are often a reality of life. Because in extended or step families, children are often absorbing two or three types of reactions, philosophies and emotions.

It is important to bear this in mind when their reactions or comments are a total mystery, beyond your understanding. They are confused. They are hurting. They are scared. They are probably feeling guilty for any variety of reasons. And equally probable, they may not be getting the positive emotional support or understanding they need in the other household during this time.

There's little you can do about any of this. Be available if they do want to talk. Encourage them to visit. And try not to worry about something you can't change.

I particularly like this piece of philosophy from Hugh Prather's book, *I Touch the Earth, the Earth Touches Me*:

> My day has become a fraction happier since I realized that nothing is exactly the way I would like it to be. This is simply a fact of life—and there goes one battle I don't have to fight anymore.

The situation with the Kwan family was totally different. Although a true-life experience, it could almost be used as a textbook example of how to handle terminal illness with youngsters.

Mr. Kwan spent hours talking with me when he learned I was writing this book and that I was concerned about dealing with children in this situation. He and his wife had two children. They were aged seven and eight when they received his wife's cancer diagnosis and eight and nine at the time she died. I admired tremendously the way they dealt with the illness.

Mr. Kwan felt that there were two basic requirements in dealing with children and cancer: Be honest with the children and remember that their security is a critical issue. His philosophy was one of the best I've ever been exposed to, not only for children but for adults as well: "In the case of a life-threatening illness, overall life is interrupted, but daily life continues."

The Kwans were on a three day ferry trip, halfway between Juneau, Alaska and Seattle, Washington, to begin a long awaited vacation for the family when Mr. Kwan received a call from their local doctor on the ship to shore radio. He was given the diagnosis concerning his wife and told that the University of Washington hospital was waiting for her to check in the day after they docked.

Mrs. Kwan was not told of the diagnosis until after she was hospitalized. The children were with them when the doctor explained that she had cancer and they were aware of her reactions, shock, concern and finally acceptance. Mr. and Mrs. Kwan included the children in the discussion of the treatments available and the possible side effects and the prognosis. The doctor promptly answered the children's questions.

Mr. Kwan made arrangements for the children to see movies showing cancer patients and some of the treatments and the ways in which the disease may progress. Without being negative or fatalistic, he wanted the children to be aware that their mother would go through some physical changes and that this was normal for the disease. Seeing other people change prepared them for the changes possible in their mother. Nurses were asked to answer questions from the children after they saw the movies.

The Kwan family remained in Seattle for the next eight months while Mrs. Kwan received cancer treatment which was unavailable in Juneau. While Mr Kwan and many clinical experts generally feel that the fewer changes the better, the situation obviously called for lifestyle changes for the Kwan family.

Initially there was no real pattern to their life in Seattle and Mr. Kwan soon realized this was bad for the children. His sister-in-law came and stayed with them in an apartment near the hospital. This provided the children with a sense of security and comfort. A pattern was soon established and the resulting routine normalized somewhat the process of dealing with their mother's illness.

The children attended school in Seattle. Mr. Kwan picked them up from school and went home with them to prepare dinner and complete any homework. They then went to the hospital to spend a half hour with their mother. His sister-in-law took the children home while he remained with Mrs. Kwan. On Saturdays, friends and family visited with Mrs. Kwan. This was the day that Mr. Kwan devoted entirely to the children, doing whatever they wanted to do, with a mid-day visit to their mother. Quality time was very important to the Kwan family.

Naturally the children would have preferred to return home to Juneau where they had many friends and a safe, well-known life. The Kwans explained that while it would be nicest to return to Juneau, they must all stay in Seattle for a while. They were honest about the fact that while the doctors might not be able to make Mom well, Seattle was the best place to try and make her better. The children were involved in the responsibility of Mom's illness and treatment. Mr. and Mrs. Kwan were very honest with the children and encouraged them to talk about any questions or concerns they had, whether it concerned their mother, their school or life in general.

Throughout the Kwan's battle with cancer, they were open and honest with the children. Children have lots of questions, such as "Do we have to go away?" "Are you going to leave us too?" "Did this happen because of something I did?" If children can't ask these questions, they will inevitably come up with the wrong answers.

When children ask questions you don't have the answers to, tell them you don't know, but will try to find out. Then get them answers.

Children are not babies, they are little people. If they are dealt with honestly and openly, they are generally able to cope with changes and crises. A child has the right to know about anything that is going to have a major effect on his or her life and cause major changes in the family's life. It may be necessary to establish new normal patterns and responsibilities. One parent cannot do it all no matter how hard they try. Explain and discuss the new responsibilities that must be shared because the sick parent can no longer do some things. Then make it clear that everyone has additional duties. Involve the children in the decision-making process instead of simply dictating new rules or decisions. Remember that they are just as concerned about Mom or Dad as you are and they are probably concerned about you too and anxious to do whatever they can.

While it is true that there will be extra responsibilities for everyone, from taking out the garbage to helping keep the house clean, it is also important that the children be encouraged to continue their lives with all the normal amounts of fun and laughter possible. Again, the premise is that life goes on and that the illness is a temporary interruption for the cancer patient and family.

If the children want to visit friends, go to sleep-overs, stay involved in their regular activities, encourage them.

Since it is impossible to do everything, this is an excellent opportunity for you to take advantage of offers of help from friends, family, hospice volunteers and so forth. These people can provide chauffeur service for the children or perhaps sit with your spouse while you attend a special event with the child. There will of course be times when the children will want to do things that just aren't possible at the moment. Do your best to offer alternatives. At one point Mr. Kwan's daughter wanted desperately to go home to Juneau. While that wasn't possible, he did offer the alternative of her calling her best friend and talking with her on the phone in private as a means of making the continued stay in Seattle easier.

Children need support and love at this time just as you do. Let the kids pick their level of involvement and their comfort level, but be sure they know they're welcome to help. If the illness has caused some major life style changes or postponement of promised events, be sure they understand that this is only an interruption or postponement. Never break a promise. In the case of the Kwan family, the diagnosis interrupted a long awaited family vacation including Disneyland. After Mrs. Kwan died, Mr. Kwan took the children on that vacation.

Create good times as often as possible throughout the illness. This is particularly important for youngsters. The Kwan family would have "Welcome Home" parties when Mrs. Kwan came home from lengthy hospital stays. The parties were complete with streamers and balloons and special treats the children would help bake. When Mrs. Kwan was unable to come home for special occasions, such as birthdays or other holidays, the family made arrangements with the hospital to take the party to her. After her death, the ability to remember and talk about the good times they'd had in spite of the illness, made accepting her death and continuing with their lives easier.

The most critical issue in dealing with young children and a parent's terminal illness depends upon the cooperation of the doctors and nurses involved. Never let the children see their parent in pain. Be sure that doctors and nurses are aware that you want the pain controlled at all times when the children are present. If necessary, rearrange the visiting schedule to be sure the parent is comfortable when the children visit the hospital.

Note to parents: Please do not attempt to titrate medication at home with the children there. It can be frightening and unsettling for adults, let alone youngsters.

Mr. Kwan feels, and I agree, that when pain can no longer be continuously controlled at home, it is better for the patient to be in the hospital or in a hospice facility. If the decision is made to keep the cancer patient at home, the alternative is for the children to stay with relatives and visit the parent.

No one can tell you what is best for you and your children. No one can tell you how you should or ought to deal with the situation. I pass along Mr. Kwan's suggestions only because they were very successful in helping his family deal with the illness. His rules were:

1. Be honest and up front with the children.
2. Involve the children in the diagnosis, decisions, responsibilities and emotions of the illness.
3. Encourage the children to continue with as normal a schedule as possible, under existing circumstances. Remember, the illness is merely an interruption of their lives and yours.
4. Never allow the children to see the parent in pain.
5. Involve the children in the problem; don't encourage them to ignore or run away from this very real part of their lives.

8

The Medical Team

SEPTEMBER 4TH -

I couldn't believe it. The doctor sat between us and, after telling us of the test results, had tears in his eyes as he put an arm around each of us and whispered, "I'm so sorry."

Our odds are one in three. If the chemo combination works, Walt could be back on his feet in less than a year. If it doesn't work, the doctor says we're looking at a few weeks to a few months.

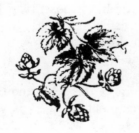

Generations past, Confucius said, "Ignorance is the night of the mind, a night without moon or star." I encourage you to learn all you can and get as much information as possible on the type of cancer your loved one is battling. Any knowledge you can obtain helps you understand what is going on and enables you to help in the treatment process. You will be spending more time with the patient than the doctors. Your insights and observations may help them in making decisions or recommendations on treatment and medication.

There is, unfortunately, a vast lack of information on many types of cancer, but at least try. If there is an American Cancer Society office in your area, they usually have a library of free pamphlets, describing the various types of cancer, the causes, effects and treatments available. Often hospice and the Visiting Nurses Association have booklets of the same type.

Explain to your specialists how much you want to know. I wanted to know the odds, the treatment, what to expect from the treatment, as well as what to expect as the disease progressed or Walt's cancer went into remission and entered the healing stages.

The amount of knowledge wanted or needed is a personal decision, differing from person to person. Even you and your loved one may want different types or levels of knowledge.

As a general rule, physicians need to be encouraged to provide you with information, particularly if it is negative information. Most people don't want to hear bad news and most physicians don't want to give bad news. Remember that the term 'physician' is culturally translated as 'healer'—one who fixes and makes well.

Most physicians will honestly answer questions and provide information if they know that is your desire.

In Shelly's case, she and David were both fully aware of the possibilities and ramifications of any proposed treatment. Dave dealt with his cancer straight on. They went to every conference and to every chemotherapy session together. Dave wanted them both to know how he was progressing. They both wanted to understand and discuss treatment options.

Dave had two goals he hoped to achieve in treatment. Since cure was not an immediate option, he wanted to lead as normal a life as possible and maintain his control over the cancer until a cure could be found. These two goals were ever present in discussions with his doctors and decisions in treatments.

Shelly and David always asked for all of the options available, any possible side effects, which treatment was the most usual route and which option the doctor would recommend. Many times they did not make an immediate decision, but took the information home and talked about it further. When a decision had been reached that both felt comfortable with, they would go back to the doctor.

In our case, Walt and I went to every conference and chemotherapy session together. Our doctors would tell us as much as Walt wanted to know. I would then call or meet with the doctors later to go over any additional questions I had or any concerns about Walt's well being. I always asked for any additional information I needed to provide the best possible care at home.

Your loved one may not want to know all the details about their treatment or progress. This is often a case of ignorance being bliss, as with Walt. I was the one wanting and needing the information. My husband had always been an expert at confrontation avoidance and often felt that what he didn't know wouldn't hurt him. My personality, conversely, dictates gathering any and all available information and preparing options for dealing with possible upcoming situations. I am most comfortable when I feel I have a handle on things, perhaps because it gives me a feeling of some control. I needed to be prepared for the positive and negative aspects of the disease, the treatments, the prognosis and the interim periods.

For some patients, not knowing may be more frightening than hearing the facts. If your loved one has questions, concerns or wants more information than you are ready to deal with, encourage him or her to talk with the doctor.

If you or your loved one don't come right out and ask, the odds are good no one is going to tell you. I learned this when I didn't ask specific questions of our oncologist in Seattle before returning home to Alaska. I simply assumed that the waiting period to see if the chemotherapy would work was going to be a quiet period of status quo. As one thing after another began going wrong, I finally called Seattle, asked the questions, got the answers and was prepared to deal with the final weeks of Walt's illness.

It is essential that you be comfortable with your doctors and specialists. They quite literally hold your loved one's life in their hands when it comes to diagnosis and treatment.

Doctors

Be up front with your doctors. Let them know how much you want to know and how involved you want to be in the treatment decision process. The more open you are with them, the easier it is for them to help you.

Can your doctor tell you where you can get the best treatment and recommend specialists or at least tell you where to find this information? Do you know of anyone in your area facing the same battle? Cancer makes friends of unknown faces dealing with the same problems.

When Walt first got sick, our family doctor was in Seattle having surgery himself and we were assigned the doctor on call at the emergency room. He diagnosed pneumonia and referred us to one of our family doctor's back-up physicians. We were not initially impressed with this doctor and after two visits over a period of three weeks when he did nothing but renew the antibiotic prescription, we changed doctors.

The new doctor immediately ordered tests done and diagnosed the cancer within three days. The decision to change doctors or specialists is your right. You are dealing with enough unknowns and anxieties. You want, need and deserve a team that works well together toward a common goal.

For this reason, don't feel you must stay with a doctor you are uncomfortable with. If you do not have a family doctor, don't feel you must take just anyone. Talk to friends about their doctors and their experiences. If you know of anyone in your area who has dealt with cancer, call them. With few exceptions, those of us who have been there are willing and anxious to offer any information and assistance we can. You might also check with the American Cancer Society or hospice for oncologists in your area.

Our friends Dave and Shelly relocated several times during their marriage and were frequently looking for and establishing new doctor-patient relationships during Dave's extended battle with lymphatic cancer. Dave's first visit with a new doctor included providing a complete medical history and a frank discussion of qualifications, billing policies and the doctor's philosophy towards treatment. Dave let the physician know that he wanted all of the medical facts and that he would be making the treatment decisions. Few doctors had any problem dealing with his no-nonsense way of working with them.

Your regular doctor will generally be the one to recommend an oncologist at a cancer center. I told our doctor I wanted to ask Shelly about Dave's oncologist in Seattle. I knew they considered him excellent. Ironically, our local doctor had studied under this same oncologist. There was a good working relationship and a feeling of real comfort on our part.

Start logging all visits to doctors. You may want to take notes during some office visits. As more physicians are brought in, it gets confusing as to whom you saw, when, what was discussed, and what treatment if any was recommended or administered. This log enables you to assist in tracking progress and identifying potential problems. Encourage communication between the physicians. Your log helps assure that today's doctor knows what yesterday's doctor said or did.

Please understand that this is not easy for your doctor either. I say this whether you are dealing with a family physician you have known for years or with a new doctor you have just met.

Dr. Charles A. Garfield, founder and director of the Shanti Project, points out in *The Impact of Death on the Health-Care Professional,*

Early in my work, I learned the difficulty inherent in the physician's role. Culturally defined as a healer, he may be forced to resort to an extreme psychological defensive posture, in order to deny the reality of many of the situations in which he works... For a culturally defined healer, death is tantamount to failure, and the emotional consequences for the physician are often severe.

Our new doctor was unknown to us prior to Walt's illness. When the test results came back, he came into Walt's room and closed the door. Sitting down on the side of the bed with us he said, "There's no easy way to say this, particularly to two young people like you. The tests indicate clearly we are dealing with lung cancer." With tears in his eyes, he put an arm around each of us, hugged us, and assured us he would do all he could to help us every step of the way.

He was out of town when Walt died. Immediately upon his return, he called me to see how I was. We always felt that we were a team with this doctor, all of us working together towards a common goal.

I include this insight to help you understand the necessity of being open with your doctor about your need or desire for information. It can't be easy for one who is trained in healing to deal with the fact that a cure may not be an option in all instances. Help your doctor to help you by letting him know you have accepted the fact that he is not a miracle worker.

Nutritionist

Ask to talk with the staff nutritionist at the hospital, a specialist in matters of calorie and protein intake. Request any help she may be able to give in attaining the nutritional level necessary for your loved one's comfort and recovery. In most cases there are some definite dietary requirements during treatment and recuperation and the nutritionist can help you design menus to meet these needs and answer the many question you may have.

The nutritionist may also be able to prepare you for possible changes in the patient's eating habits. For example, many patients develop a strong dislike of red meats after chemotherapy. Walt had always had a very active sweet tooth, but after a couple of chemotherapy treatments he had no desire at all for the cookies and candy people brought over to help reach his required calorie intake. The nutritionist should be able to provide recipes and suggestions for tempting your loved one's appetite and making the required dietary changes or additions at least palatable. The American Cancer Society also has booklets available for dealing with the requirements and changing tastes of cancer patients.

Nurses

Talk with the nurses. Nurses in cancer wards are among the most caring and helpful individuals I have ever met. Often they have practical tips and advice from their experience with cancer. They can answer questions and provide a great deal of help in preparing to care for your spouse at home.

While we did not have a cancer ward at our local hospital, the nurses were just as wonderful. Knowing my concerns, they would advise me of any changes that had occurred while I was gone from the hospital. They were always ready to answer any questions I had and make suggestions for Walt's comfort or making things easier for me when we returned home. Don't be afraid to ask for their help and suggestions. They want to help if you'll let them know that it is welcome.

9
Getting Help

...Following the nurses' suggestion, I asked security for an escort and he walked me back to the hotel—it was pleasant not to have to wait around for a cab, scurry out of the hospital, ride three blocks and scurry into the hotel. Seems this is one of the services the hospital provides patients' families and hospital staff, if they live/park within certain parameters.

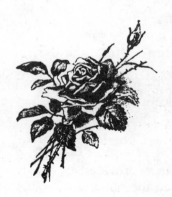

Things move so fast. You're trying to understand what is happening, learn as much as possible from your doctor, make decisions on specialists and where to go for treatment, possibly make travel arrangements, find someone to keep the kids, feed the dog and watch the house. In addition, a part of you recognizes that this represents huge expenses in potential travel, hotels, hospital bills, drugs and other medical assistance, all at a time when you are obviously losing one or more incomes. It seems inevitable that Murphy's Law swings into action: "If anything can go wrong, it will and at the worst possible time." Be prepared for it.

The chapter, "Friends and Relatives", is a solid reminder to you of the things that other people can do to free your time for your loved one and yourself. This is the time to accept and encourage any and all legitimate offers of assistance!

1. *Call the American Cancer Society (ACS) in your area.*

The assistance provided by local chapters may vary depending upon the number of volunteers and the funds available. In our instance, they covered three hundred dollars of travel expenses for required out of town treatment in each fiscal year. Since the round trip air fare to the nearest cancer center was four hundred ninety-five dollars per person, this was a big help. My friend Shelly on the other hand, had never been told this assistance was available when her husband David had to go to Seattle on various occasions for treatment.

The local ACS may work with the local Easter Seals, hospice, Visiting Nurses Associations and other organizations to provide necessary sick room equipment. Through this effort we were able to get a hospital bed and an oxygen condenser. Without the condenser, a three thousand dollar piece of equipment, we would have been unable to bring Walt home, as he used the equivalent of one tank of oxygen every two hours. If you cannot locate a local ACS, contact their national office at (404) 320-3333.

Some ACS agencies provide Ensure, a nutritional supplement, to the cancer patient free of charge and provide delivery as well. The practical importance of Ensure is discussed in the chapter on "Home Nursing." In our case, we had to make arrangements with the research hospital in Seattle to provide the Ensure. A friend's mother picked up several cases at a time and another friend, who worked on the ferry system, brought the Ensure from Seattle to Juneau as part of his personal luggage allotment. Had we purchased the Ensure from the local drug store, the cost was approximately ten dollars for a six pack of three ounce cans! We were receiving it from the institute by the case. This was a classic case of Ask for Help that involved a network of people, some of whom we'd met only once.

Check with the American Cancer Society, either where you live or where you are taking treatment, to see if they provide the "I Can Cope" series for cancer families. This series addresses all areas of cancer treatment and care as well as the emotional issues you may be dealing with. You will meet some wonderful people who are dealing with a situation similar to yours.

In many areas, the ACS provides the CanSurmount Patient Visitor Program, which offers emotional support and information to the cancer victim and the family. CanSurmount volunteers are cancer patients themselves. They have been right where you are and can provide a valuable support system as well as assistance in locating services you may need.

If you have to go to another city for diagnosis, tests or treatment, get in touch with the ACS there. You will generally find that cities with cancer centers have a very active group to help out-of-town families with the practical issues that can be so frustrating and so expensive at this time.

We had to go to Seattle, the nearest center for cancer diagnosis, testing and treatment. I called ACS there. ACS had agreements with several hotels to provide complimentary rooms to cancer victims and their families. We were in Seattle for twelve days and paid only for meals and telephone calls, while staying at comfortable, friendly hotels. There is no way of describing the relief of not having to worry about reservations in an unknown town or a thousand-dollar-plus hotel bill at the end of treatment. Our hotels were within walking distance of the hospital, which was marvelous, as I could get some exercise and fresh air to balance the ten to twelve hours spent each day in Walt's hospital room.

2. *Call the hospital.*

If your spouse is hospitalized, check with the hospital for any services they provide families of cancer patients. At Swedish Hospital in Seattle, there were many services available to make our stay easier. Their Social Services agency provided information on Seattle American Cancer Society services, other agencies that might provide assistance, local bus routes and shopping facilities, and gave us several helpful booklets. The hospital provided a separate lounge where families could chat with visitors without disturbing the patient or where spouses could nap during the night if necessary. On days that I didn't leave for meals, because of treatment or because Walt was restless, I was usually able to order meals for myself. And, very important to me, the hospital security guards were available as escorts after dark to the parking lot or to the hotel if it was within walking distance.

There are many people out there anxious to help. Don't hesitate to ask.

3. *Call the local Social Security Office.*

If your loved one is eligible for Social Security at retirement, he or she is probably eligible for Social Security disability benefits. Filing with Social Security needs to be done as soon as possible. There is a five month waiting period for disability benefits and that five months is based on the date the claim is filed, not the date the illness begins.

Depending on Social Security staffing levels and office policy, you may be able to describe your situation and complete a major portion of the forms over the telephone. If not, ask them to mail the required forms or to prepare a package for someone to pick up.

Be prepared to fill out seemingly unending pages of forms, containing questions that appear to have no apparent relevance to anything. Information gathering is a prerequisite to verification of your needs with any government agency. Make copies of any form you send to anyone. I was frequently faced with calls that a form had

been misplaced or never received. Several times I was
called for verification or clarification of a response. At this
point in time you will probably find that your memory is
even shorter than your patience where paperwork is concerned and being able to refer to a copy of your original
response is tremendously helpful.

In the event that the illness almost totally eliminates
the family's income, there is a supplemental program
available from Social Security to assist during the five
month waiting period. Application for this program
requires establishing "need".

Depending upon the personality of the staff member
you draw, this can be an encouraging or discouraging
process. In my case, it was tremendously frustrating.
Social Security seemed to require "just one more form",
questioned the validity of most estimates, required letters
from our bank and generally managed to make me feel
like some sort of social parasite. Just hang in there with
clenched teeth, fill out their forms and answer their questions. The critical issue is getting your spouse well cared
for and comfortable while paying the bills. Go after all
the help you need.

On a brighter note, a close friend applied for disability when her husband recently suffered a stroke. She had
none of my negative experiences, only piles of forms to
be completed.

Whenever you talk with anyone at Social Security, or
any other agency, make a note of that person's name in
your trusty notebook. If you have questions, it is much
easier to talk with your original contact than to have to
explain the situation all over again. If you receive calls for
the same or additional information from another individual in the agency, you can refer them to your original contact.

Explain your situation clearly and carefully to the Social Security office, the illness, the diagnosis, income concerns, expense concerns, insurance coverage. If given a complete picture, they may be aware of other local, state and federal programs which can be of assistance. If they don't propose additional agencies to contact, ask if they are aware of any additional agencies or programs you might contact. At any time during or after the illness you may need financial assistance, home nursing help or domestic help. It's easier to have information you don't use than to need information you don't have.

Needless to say, list all suggested agencies or programs in the notebook you bought as suggested in the First Week Checklist in Appendix A.

4. *Check with the Veteran's Administration (VA).*

If your loved one is a veteran, the VA is another source of potential assistance. Most veterans with service related disabilities are familiar with their benefits. However, certain benefits are available to all veterans. With the constant changes occurring in the VA policies and procedures, it is best to call and clarify what assistance is currently available under your particular set of circumstances.

Start checking as soon as possible on available veteran's benefits. Again, there is a waiting period while the paperwork is processed. Be prepared for lots of paperwork and realize that processing the completed paperwork may take months.

Whether your loved one was in Vietnam or not, I found a wealth of information in the Viet Vet Survival Guide (Ballantine Books 1985).

If there is no VA hospital in your area, check to see if the VA has contracted with one of the local hospitals to provide medical services. Our closest VA hospital was two thousand miles away by air. Local hospital expenses were treated as if they were VA hospital expenses by the Veteran's Administration and the VA paid any bills not covered by our insurance.

In these instances, the VA works on a pre-authorization basis. When you check into the hospital, be sure to tell the check-in desk your loved one is a veteran. Advise doctors, hospice, anyone who may bill you for services. We had to get pre-authorization for the oxygen tanks and equipment, as well as for hospital stays, hospice care and physician visits. Most medical agencies know what to do if the patent is a veteran, but you must tell them of the veteran status. Pre-authorization is critical to assure timely payments by the VA.

Try to have a copy of the vet's DD214, a standard military form, available as well as their service number. It seems the VA cannot function without these two items. In the event there is no DD214 easily found , contact the VA office in the city where the veteran was discharged. They should be able to get a copy for you.

A word of caution: If your doctor or oncologist sends you to a cancer center (such as our treatment at Swedish Hospital in Seattle) where there is also a VA hospital, you will receive no VA assistance with bills from the cancer center.

Our oncologist worked with Swedish Hospital. Swedish had an entire floor devoted to the care and treatment of cancer patients. The Seattle VA had no such accommodations and to the best of my knowledge, based on telephone conversations with the regional VA office, had no oncologist on staff. However, since there was a VA hospital in Seattle, Walt could have been "made comfortable" at the VA, with no expense to us. If we went to

Swedish Hospital, where he could receive the best in diagnostic testing and treatment, the VA could offer no financial help. Quite frankly, Walt was more important to me than their free hospital room with no specialized assistance for cancer.

5. *Call any agencies recommended to you by others.*

This is not the time to be a proud person, which is part of what makes coping with the illness so traumatic for most of us. As independent individuals, it is much easier to give than to receive, much easier to offer help than to ask for it. Asking for and accepting assistance were among the hardest things I had to learn.

There are a number of agencies and programs willing and able to help folks just like us. Give them a chance to be givers. Don't hesitate to contact any agency that can make life easier for you and your loved one.

10

Home Versus Hospital

-October 18th -

Herb, Chuck, Preston and I picked up the oxygen condenser and hospital bed from the Easter Seals warehouse and I picked Walt up at the hospital at 7:00. We had a short "celebration party" and Walt was in bed by 10:00. Chuck and Penny stayed and I had a short, healing cry. They left and I contemplated what the next few weeks and months would bring.

With new technology, equipment and services available, more and more cancer patients are offered the option of returning to their own homes. Until a few years ago, the only choice for those facing terminal illness was usually weeks of hospitalization. The emergence of hospice and home health care organizations has been the key to making home a practical alternative. However, don't for a minute believe it is going to be an easy or simple alternative.

There are tremendous advantages and rewards attached to being able to spend this time with your loved one. There are also tremendous responsibilities involved. The decision is one that will need to be made by a team, including your doctor and the health care professionals in your area. You, the loved one and caregiver, need to vote too. This is not a decision to be made merely because you think you "should" do something. And the decision may change from time to time. I wanted Walt home. Walt wanted to be at home. We could talk and watch television together on his good days. I had a feeling about the length of time we had together and, therefore, the more time the better. But, full-time nursing of someone you love is very trying, to say the least. It can be a tremendous strain, physically, mentally and emotionally.

Full time nursing is exactly what you may be facing. After we brought Walt home, I was a full time, twenty-four hour a day, on-call nurse. Our case was perhaps somewhat unique in that he required a high level of oxygen and Juneau is infamous for power outages year round, but especially fall and winter, the seasons we were dealing with. If the power went out, he had to switch immediately to a portable oxygen cylinder. Because he spent so much time napping, and might not be aware of a power outage, leaving him alone at the house was not a viable option.

There were medications to administer and reactions to be monitored and noted; the last month he was taking Demerol injections, which I administered. The hospice nurses were terrific, but they couldn't be there every time something needed to be done.

None of this is said to discourage you. Although I had no idea what home care was going to involve, I'd do it all over again, now that I've been educated. I would, however, do some of it differently. Primarily, I would ask for more help and treat myself better.

The last time we put Walt in the hospital, it was to try to level out the medications we had been titrating at home and find a comfort level for him. At the same time, the hospice nurse and the emergency room doctor made it very clear that it was also necessary for my sake that he spend a couple of days in the hospital. I had had no more than a couple of hours sleep at any one time over a period of six days and was not in very good shape myself.

Each individual must acknowledge their human limits and their emotional limits. I read once that there is little difference between keeping your chin up and sticking out your neck. In this case, it's important to know what that difference is. It's not easy to see your loved one in pain or discomfort, knowing that you can do nothing further to help. Intellectually, you recognize that they could do no more for your loved one if he was in the hospital but here at home you may feel somehow responsible, frustrated and helpless. At one time or another, I experienced all of these emotions plus moments of resentment and exhaustion. However, we had so many good moments out of that period of time that these negative emotions passed quickly.

The single most difficult issue for me to deal with was the full-time, day and night exposure to Walt's discomfort, whether waking or sleeping. The single most positive issue was being there for each other, regardless of the time of day or night.

There are lots of negatives, and just as many payoffs, to having your loved one at home throughout the difficult phases of a terminal illness. There are several questions to be answered in making the decision:

- Does your loved one want to be at home?
- Are you physically able to care for the patient?
- Are you emotionally able to care for the patient?
- Does the doctor agree this is an option?
- Can you get nursing or domestic help, if needed?
- Are you personally ready to nurse your loved one?

If responses to the above are "Yes", get as much information as you can to help make the final decision.

First talk with your doctor about what kind of care will be required. Will any special equipment be necessary? Can he help make arrangements to get that equipment? Are there public or private agencies that can assist?

When the hospice or the Visiting Nurses Association is involved, talk next with one of their nurses. They are, in my opinion, the greatest resource available for anyone considering home care for a terminal illness. Their experience and expertise allow them to honestly answer your questions and concerns, outline just what is involved and offer practical help and suggestions.

Armed with all the facts, hopefully you and your loved one can make as objective a decision as is possible in these circumstances. Bear in mind that a forced or unwilling decision to have your loved one at home, with around the clock nursing responsibility, can lead to resentment, physical and emotional deterioration and bad feelings about yourself that do nothing positive for any of the parties involved. Also be aware that either of you have the right to change your decision at any time. If there is a hospice facility in your area, this is an excellent alternative, one that provides a homelike atmosphere but does not require twenty-four hour nursing on your part and solves the problem of pain control where there are children involved.

Recognize that your Yes or No response to home care may change as circumstances change. I said "yes" overall. However, after three days, I had to say "no" to completing the titrating at home. Two weeks later when they prescribed intravenous morphine injections for the pain, I again had to say "no". Knowing that a miscalculation could result in Walt's death, I was unwilling and emotionally unable to accept that responsibility. We were very fortunate that a friend was a registered nurse and agreed to stay at the house the first night until we could locate a private-duty nurse.

The book, *Why Die (Live) at Home?* by John D. Muir, presents the following list of advantages for home as an alternative to the hospital:

1. It's natural.
2. The patient can influence quality and quantity of his/her own life.
3. Respect and dignity are maintained.
4. The patient feels wanted.
5. You feel useful and needed.
6. The continued presence of a loved one supports you both.
7. You can both live more normally and fully.
8. You can both have more freedom and control. No one will wake your spouse at five-thirty in the morning to take his/her temperature.
9. There is time and a place to deal with the feelings of love, anger and grief.
10. No travel wear and tear between home and hospital, no worry about loved ones driving on bad roads.
11. You can see and create your own version of beauty, not institutional green walls.
12. You can cater to the loved one's requests and desires for food.
13. Living at home costs less.
14. It's home!

Hospice

If there is a hospice organization in your area, you may not need to look any further for home health care. Not only do they provide marvelous services themselves, they are usually aware of other services available in the area. In our instance, hospice personnel knew where to go to get the hospital equipment we needed to bring Walt home.

Hospice is an organization, as well as a theory about health care. Dr. Sylvia A. Lack, a national hospice organizer, says, "The main concern of a hospice program is the management of terminal disease in such a way that the patients live until they die, that their families live with them as they are dying... and go on living afterwards."

The hospice team includes professional caregivers and volunteers who generally assist in caring for the patient in the home. The emphasis is on managing and alleviating pain and making the patient and family comfortable physically and psychologically. If you don't find a listing in the phone book, check with your doctor or call the National Hospice Organization at (703) 243-5900.

Available services vary from area to area. In Juneau, we had two registered nurses, a counselor and several volunteers at the time of Walt's illness. In Florida, where I now live, there are several hospice organizations, providing everything from visiting nurses and volunteers to a hospice facility for the patients who cannot, for whatever reason, remain in their own home but do not want to live in a hospital environment. In Juneau, the nurses saw the patient at home regularly and we had a twenty-four hour "beeper" number, should the need arise for professional assistance. Hospice may provide a program like the one we had in Juneau. It may be an organization of volunteers-only, available to help in the home; it may include a stand-alone hospice facility or it may function as an in-patient unit of the local hospital.

The counselor in Juneau visited with us once but, in all honesty, we were much more comfortable talking with each other and our pastor. Because of our large network of family and friends, we did not call upon the hospice volunteers. However, after Walt's death, I worked with the hospice organization and presented a segment of their volunteer training program. Because of this, I am very aware of the compassion, caring and sincere concern on the part of the volunteers to help the families in whatever way possible. The hospice volunteers make themselves available to run errands; help with the housework or cooking, if needed; provide periodic child care or simply stay with your spouse, so you can get out of the house and take care of you.

Although I was vaguely aware of the existence of hospice, I'd had no previous experience with the organization. When Walt had to have supplemental oxygen, he was admitted through the emergency room in the evening. Two days later, when I walked into his hospital room mid-morning, he said, "Someone named Mary was here to see us, but she said she'd come back when you were here. She left a card." Our doctor, fully aware of Walt's feeling about being in hospital for any length of time, had called hospice himself to start the process of being able to come back home.

Our hospice nurses were on call twenty-four hours a day in the event a situation came up which we couldn't deal with. The first call I placed was when Walt's pain exceeded a level that could be handled by the oral medication he was receiving. They contacted our doctor, got permission for Demoral injections and taught me how to give them. On another occasion, they simply assured me that Walt's reaction to a new medicine was not uncommon nor unexpected, and educated me on what to look for and how to deal with it.

Knowing I was interested, concerned and determined to keep Walt at home, they took the time to be sure I was aware of how to subtly take his pulse, check his respirations, monitor reactions to everything from medicine to food. I very quickly learned when to call and when not to, although there was never any impatience when I called with something that really wasn't important.

The night Walt had a major and negative reaction to one of the titrating experiences, the hospice nurse came out to the house, called the hospital and took both of us to the emergency room in her car, making sure Walt was settled and I had friends to take me home later. In addition to being on call, the nurses worked closely with our doctor and came out to the house two or three times a week, just to make sure we were okay.

The biggest problem the nurses had was me. As I've mentioned several times, I didn't take care of myself as I should have, nor did I take time off as I should have and they knew it. If there is an exception to my statement about ignoring "should and ought" requirements, I think it would be when those statements come from your hospice, Visiting Nurses Association or home health care nurses. They are as concerned about you, the caregiver, as they are about the patient.

Visiting Nurses Association (VNA)

Visiting Nurses Association (VNA), a United Way agency, also provides community-based home health care. VNA was established more than a century ago to provide licensed, non-profit care for individuals needing assistance within their homes. The assistance available may vary from area to area.

In addition to skilled nursing personnel, VNA home health aides may assist in bathing the patient, preparing meals or doing light housework. Their volunteer groups provide friendly visits to the patient or family, telephone reassurance, and adult day care centers. VNA also has live-in companions who are available around the clock, seven days a week.

Like hospice, VNA can help establish the level of assistance you need and train you to administer medications or meet special dietary needs. Like the American Cancer Society, VNA maintains Loan Closets, which can provide needed home health care equipment. VNA social workers can assist in solving financial or social problems that may occur.

In many cases, your doctor may contact the Visiting Nurses Association about your loved one's return home. Or you may call them, explain your situation and ask if they can help. A doctor's referral and the need for skilled nursing or monitoring of medication, food or side effects will establish your eligibility for VNA services.

Most VNA services are covered by Medicare, Medicaid, Veterans Administration, Worker's Compensation or private insurance. Be sure to discuss any insurance restrictions with the VNA representative. In cases where there is no insurance, or the coverage is severely restricted, United Way funding may be available to help cover the costs of the home health care requirements.

We didn't have a VNA office in Juneau at the time of Walt's illness. Therefore, I have no personal experience with their organization. However, Chris Allen, the Home Health Care Coordinator in Melbourne, Florida, provided me a great deal of information. If Chris is representative of the caring and ability of VNA staff, their organization provides the same support, skills and understanding that I found in the Juneau Hospice group.

If you don't find a VNA office listed in your local directory, contact their National Hotline, (800) 426-2547, for assistance.

Home Health Care Organizations

Since 1985, there have been a number of other home health care organizations developing across the nation. These people are caring, supportive professionals. They can answer questions, assist in obtaining equipment, explain possible side effects of medication and treatments and generally become your medical support group.

Be aware that many insurance policies now cover home health care provided by licensed and approved agencies. Our insurance covered one hundred percent of the hospice billings during Walt's illness. Some organizations do not bill patients direct or they bill based on financial circumstances. Your doctor is probably aware of the home health care assistance available in your area.

Your telephone directory may list local agencies under "nursing", "health care", or "home health care".

In addition to medical assistance, you may need help with the practical tasks of day-to-day living. This is particularly true if the cancer patient has previously taken care of the housework and cooking chores. In the event that there are no hospice or home health care volunteers in your area to help with these tasks, there may be other agencies that have domestic help available specifically for housebound invalids. For instance, Kelly Girls now has a home care division, geared to assisting in such circumstances. Be sure to clarify whether or not agency services are covered by insurance, if this is a specific concern.

Again, ask your doctor, your friends, your support group, and your telephone directory for help.

11
Home Nursing

-OCTOBER 23RD -

The doctor advised us today he wants x-rays to see if the tumor is advancing. Walt couldn't sleep. Called the hospice at 9:30 about doubling up on pain medication. Judy came out, gave him a Demoral injection, taught me how to give one and left syringes. I am not looking forward to the first time I give Walt an injection.

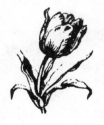

I f you have decided that your loved one is going to remain at home, there are a number of practical hints to make it easier. In addition to the suggestions included here, check with your hospice or home health care organization for services and references they can supply. They may also have helpful booklets available.

Equipment

Medical and hospital-type equipment may be a major consideration. In our case, we got a hospital bed to assure Walt's ability to sit up for ease of breathing. However, the most important piece of equipment in our case was an oxygen condenser, required because of Walt's extremely high oxygen level usage. The hospital bed could have been rented, had there been an equipment rental facility in town. The oxygen condenser however, was a delicate, highly technical piece of equipment and very expensive.

In Sue's case, a shower chair and walker were needed for John to function at home. They discovered that almost any home health care equipment can be rented or may be made available through organizations such as American Cancer Society, Visiting Nurses Association or the

Easter Seals agency. Ask your doctor if you have no idea where to start.

The use of any hospital type equipment should, as much as possible, be left up to the patient. We had a hospital bed for Walt, as he frequently had trouble breathing before he went on the oxygen. Additionally, with all the naps he needed, there were more choices of position. The hospital bed was set up in our bedroom which fortunately was large enough for both it and our queen sized bed. He used the hospital bed only two nights. To him it was very simple, "I didn't marry you to lay over there and watch you sleep alone!" We did keep it throughout the illness, as an option for comfort, but he never used it again. The very night he died, when I asked if he wanted to go back and lay down for a while, he said, "Yes, as long as I can get in my own bed."

Diet and Calories for the Patient

Most cancer patients have very high calorie and protein requirements. At the same time, they have finicky appetites, if they're hungry at all. Chemotherapy often causes nausea. Fortunately there are several medications available to reduce or eliminate this particular side effect of treatment.

Often a person's tastes and preferences will change drastically as a result of chemotherapy or radiation treatment. Confirmed steak eaters may literally get nauseous at the sight of red meat. Dedicated shellfish lovers may get violently ill when faced with shrimp fettucini. Be prepared for this. You may find that you suddenly have a spouse or loved one who wants omelets, cheese casseroles and baked flounder. You will probably begin to understand my strong positive feelings about Ensure milk shakes. Roll with the punches and try to gauge your spouse's reactions to various foods. Then keep acceptable snacks available for the patient.

One of the greatest sources of calorie and protein is a product called Ensure, sold in most drug stores and usually available through cancer centers. A single can of Ensure contains three hundred fifty calories. When that is mixed in the blender with an egg, maybe some milk and a scoop of ice cream, you can really bring the calorie count up. There were days when this was the only thing Walt could get down and he did that by sheer willpower.

Get yourself a calorie book, the kind you usually buy to determine what you can't eat in the interest of losing weight! Read it from right to left with pencil in hand, underlining or highlighting those items with the highest calorie content. This is your guide to menu planning. I used *LeGette's Calorie Encyclopedia* by Bernard LeGette since it included fast foods, frozen foods, home cooked meals and snacks.

Fortunately Walt continued to enjoy lots of high calorie foods, fried rice, milk shakes, lasagna, etc. But he lost all desire for high calorie desserts such as cakes, pies and cookies. One of the biggest frustrations you may face is fixing high calorie meals, knowing these will provide the daily calorie requirement, and then accepting the fact that your loved one simply cannot eat the meal.

Do the best you can. Continue to tempt the patient but try not to nag. This is a tough piece of advice to follow. You're trying to do everything you can to meet the suggestions of the doctors and the nutritionist and some days it seems your loved one just isn't interested in cooperating!

Walt always ate better at home than when he was in the hospital. Probably because his favorites were generally available and he could eat when he was hungry, not when a meal was scheduled. One time while he was in the hospital, I was encouraging him to at least try to eat more of his dinner. He finally looked at me and said, "I'd eat if I was hungry or thought any of this would stay down. I've done the best I could. Would you just get off my back!"

As far as Walt was concerned, I wasn't encouraging, I was nagging, and it wasn't what he needed at the time. There is a fine line between encouragement and nagging. Just do your best to recognize when you are close to crossing over it.

Record Keeping/Medicine

There is an immediate need for keeping track of details. If your loved one was in the hospital, the nurses would be making notes on the chart at the bed. This type of record keeping is now your responsibility. The sooner you start keeping track of what's going on, the better.

Hopefully, you've already got your notebook, with information on doctor's visits and such. If so, this now becomes your home tracking system as well. Usually you are provided with a "med chart" by the visiting nurses. If not, perhaps you can use the chart in the back of this book, having a friend make copies or simply making one up by hand.

It is important to note what medication was given and when for several reasons. First, if the patient is complaining of pain, you may not remember just when they had their last pain pill or injection. Recording medications given tells you that either it's time for more medication or that the current medication is not sufficient to keep them comfortable for the prescribed amount of time. If there are side effects, such as headaches or nausea, it is very helpful if the doctor or nurse can see a tie in to a specific

medication. In Walt's case, one of the medications for respiratory relief caused blinding headaches. After three days
of consistent reaction, our doctor was able to determine
the cause of the headaches and prescribe another type of
respiratory medication.

Med charts become critical if you begin titrating medication. We were offered the alternative of titrating at
home or in the hospital. In retrospect, I should have cho-
sen the hospital.

Titrating is the process of experimenting with different amounts and combinations of various medications to
find a point at which the patient is not is pain but is still
functional. We were not successful doing this at the
house, but a part of that was due to the unknown rapid
advancement of the tumor in the lung.

In just the past few years, technology and equipment
has changed and advanced in so many ways, that titrating
of pain medication is not near the struggle we faced. All
the pain medications, with the exception of the Demoral
injections, were given orally in pill form. When this is the
case, it takes time for the pill to work through the
patient's system and actually reduce the pain. Oral pain
medications today are tremendously effective if the
patient has not been in extreme pain for long periods of
time. In most cases, pain can be controlled at home right
up to the end. Many pain medications can now be given
through intravenous (IV) methods which provide for
almost instant relief. IV systems can be installed in the
home and your hospice or VNA nurse can show you how
to monitor the medication. If extreme pain is not an
issue, or if IV pain medications are available, titrating may
not be the task it was for us.

For days we varied between Walt being in pain and
Walt being a zombie. Finally, his respiration was so

reduced that I called the nurse and we checked into the hospital to establish medication levels. However, the chart showing what medication had occurred at what time, combined with the journal showing his reactions and my concerns were extremely helpful in being able to determine that hospitalization was needed and in assisting the doctor to decide where to start and what hadn't worked to that point.

If you need to do titrating of medications, talk with both your doctor and your home health care team about the methods that will be used, what side effects to anticipate and what the options for titrating are.

If you are the type of person who keeps any kind of diary or journal, you're way ahead of the game here. I have always kept a journal of day to day activities, thoughts, traumas, triumphs and so on. In Seattle, that journal expanded to include visits to doctors, comments on treatment at the hospital, Walt's good and bad days and his response to treatment. When we returned home, in addition to my daily journal, I added a small, three by five inch notebook and shortly thereafter the med charts provided by hospice. These all resided on the breakfast bar. In the notebook, I logged everything that Walt ate in an effort to reach the twenty-four hundred calorie per day requirement the nutritionist had given us. As time passed and complications began and medications increased, I also started noting any unusual reactions or characteristics I noticed in Walt, any increased pain levels, those occasions when he couldn't keep food down and any ideas I had about whether it might be from the chemotherapy or from a prolonged coughing spell or anything else.

Following are copies of actual pages from my notebook. You will notice that it is very simple, but towards the end it was worth its weight in gold. The initial page shows standard entries; the final page contains a great deal of not so positive information. Yet this information was critical to the hospice nurse in making the decision to move Walt back to the hospital to finish the titrating process. Our regular doctor was out of town and although we knew the back-up doctor, he hadn't been treating Walt on a day to day basis and so needed some history. The notebook provided him with much of the information he needed.

10/07/85	
Ensure w/egg	350
	72
Corn Total	270
Toast - 1	175
Coffee w/sugar I	50
Ensure w/ice cream	350
	280
Small Salad	280
Lasagna	408
Ensure	350
	2585

Down day, Walt real tired and napped a lot. Complaining of real discomfort around the lung area... talked to the doctor, but no enlightenment so far.

Severe coughing spell and lost dinner about 8:00 pm. How long does food have to stay down for the calories to be processed by the body?

10/22/85	
Ensure	350
w/1 T Molasses	143
Oatmeal, 1T Br Sugar	45
Ensure	350
Grape Juice	100
Ensure w/banana	380
	1368

10/25/85
Ensure   350

Stomach cramps across tummy, just above waist. Started about 9:30. DiGel is not helping. Tried cereal, didn't stay down. Dry heaves at 10:50. Dry heaves at 12:15.

(A call to the doctor with the above information resulted in tests that revealed an ulcer.)

11/02/85
Ensure   350
Cinnamon roll   145

Started the new medications yesterday and Walt is really groggy and acting sedated today. I am told this could last 48 hours. He is not at all hungry this morning.

Ensure   350
Scrambled Eggs (1)   100
Toast (1)   175
Ensure   350
                                                       1470

No appetite today at all. He forced himself to eat eggs but could not face supper. Slept most of the day, varying between bed and recliner. Refuses to use the hospital bed and is terribly impatient about the oxygen when awake—which is rare—and only to ask for medication. Has been asking for Demerol injections earlier than usual the last few days.

11/06/85
Ensure w/egg   350
                                                         72
Cinnamon Roll   145

Walt is still literally a zombie, in some cases bouncing off the wall when trying to walk. We have increased, decreased, spread out medication for six days and there is no leveling off. No appetite.

Ensure   350

Walt can't stay awake. He isn't even aware the Heusslers were here. He came to the table to eat supper and when I brought over my plate he was asleep sitting up. His breathing doesn't sound right.

This was the night Walt went back into the hospital so they could monitor the medications on a twenty-four hour basis. The hospice nurse and the emergency room doctor reviewed the med charts and the notebook to determine where medication caused significant changes both in requests for pain relief and Walt's ability to function. This is the point where I finally said "I can't do this. I'm not a nurse and I'm not convinced I know enough to handle all that's going on."

I should also admit that since I had not been taking care of myself, I was physically, mentally and emotionally exhausted after a week of watching my husband's condition changing like a roller coaster ride. Our hospice nurse told me quite honestly that they were putting Walt in the hospital for forty-eight hours as much for my health as for his.

If it seems like I keep saying "write it down" every other page, one of the key reasons is stress. Short term memory seemed to disappear as Walt's medical condition worsened. I couldn't remember where I had set something down two hours ago, let alone what doctor we saw on what day, what medication was administered, when we were to see what doctor again!

Night Sweats

One of the most frustrating side effects of tumor cancers is referred to as night sweats. The patient may be literally drenched in sweat several times a night and you can run yourself ragged trying to keep up with fresh bedding.

Take a page from the hospital staff's book on coping by using flannel sheets. Lay in a supply of the light weight, summer-flannel flat sheets and regular pillow cases. The sheets can be folded to the size of the upper half of the body and don't cause uncomfortable bumps and ridges if they are two or three layers thick. When night sweats occur, simply replace the flannel sheet and the pillow case. The patient doesn't have to be moved to a chair or another bed while the entire bed is changed .

Tumors often generate heat. Be prepared to wear sweaters and even jackets while your spouse is in shorts and a tee shirt, with the windows open and the outside temperature hovering at forty degrees.

The Telephone

The single biggest favor you can do yourself is to buy an answering machine of some type. There are a number of good quality machines available for under a hundred dollars. Not only is it necessary when the patient is home, in order to preserve some quiet so his or her sleep isn't disturbed, but it is often a much-needed link to the outside world.

When Walt was on medication and having trouble sleeping at night, I would unplug the phones in the back part of the house. I turned the ringer off the phone plugged into the recorder, which was placed near my favorite chair. If someone called, I would know when I heard the recorder turn on and I could talk to them without the phone disturbing Walt's rest.

When Walt was in the hospital and I was with him from ten in the morning until nine at night, it was so good to come home and find encouraging messages from friends or invitations to come out for a late dinner.

Often people are afraid to call for fear of disturbing the patient or waking you from a much needed nap. The fact that we had a recorder was common knowledge among our friends, and folks felt free to call and offer assistance, encouragement or just a friendly Hello. With the recorder functioning as a secretary, I had no hesitation in asking friends to give us a call and to keep in touch.

The recorder also meant that should we miss a call from the doctor's office, we were always aware of any test results, questions or treatment schedules.

Nursing your loved one at home requires more than your practical skills. This shared journey with all its ups and downs will not only bring you and your loved one closer together but it will call, as well, on your deepest inner resources and your capacity to care.

12

Insurance Record-Keeping

-OCTOBER 2ND -

Got three weeks worth of bills, mail and medical sorted into stacks and ready to be dealt with. Wonder if I'll ever see the surface of the breakfast bar again?

I don't care if I never see another piece of paper with blank boxes or fill-in-the-space lines.

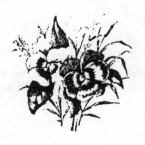

A t the point in your life when nothing makes sense and all you want to do is will your loved one back to perfect health, a practical consideration like record keeping becomes a critical issue, but one many of us are not aware of until it is too late.

Medical Insurance Claims

As soon as you have received the diagnosis, have some idea of what options you wish to pursue and can force yourself to function, get out the insurance benefits booklet(s) explaining any coverage you may have. Skim the major medical and catastrophic illness sections and then contact the insurance company. In the long run, it will make your life a lot easier if they know that they will be receiving an on-going stream of high dollar billings.

Find out if you must show a consistent single claim number in order for the billings to fall under catastrophic coverage. Most policies are written in such a manner that once you pass a specific dollar amount, regardless of the percentage of standard coverage, the insurance picks up one hundred percent of the bills. Verify this cut-off amount when you talk with your insurance representative. Also verify if this is a cut-off amount for the entire year's expenses or if you need to identify the beginning of the cancer expenses.

There are a number of things you may be able to do to make the paperwork easier to deal with and save a lot of time and hassle. The majority of hospitals, doctors, laboratories and nursing services are willing to bill your insurance carrier if they are provided with all the necessary information. Having them bill the insurance carrier directly means you are not perpetually reaching for your checkbook and reduces the amount of paperwork you have to do at home.

I always carried a copy of the original insurance claim with me. This provided our group number, Walt's claim number, the employer information and Walt's service ID number. Busy insurance clerks appreciate the fact that you are trying to help them help you.

Although it may seem to be a hassle, if it's at all possible, keep a copy of all billings you send the insurance company or anyone else. This not only makes it a lot easier to know what they are and are not paying, but is essential if there are any other benefits such as Veterans Administration payments coming. I had friends with access to copy machines and they were more than willing to respond to my requests for copies.

I kept a copy of the first claim I sent stapled to the inside front of the insurance folder so that, whenever I had to file a claim, I had Walt's employment history, group number, social security number, claim number and all the other miscellaneous information that seems to be necessary no matter how many claims you file in a week!

If you don't have access to copying capabilities, I suggest using something similar to the hand written log shown below. It's a good idea to keep a log similar to this as a quick reference, in addition to copies of claims and billings. The critical issue is establishing a simple but consistent method for keeping track of billings received, claims submitted and payments made. Medical bookkeepers and insurance clerks are not perfect. There were instances where we received bills for services that had already been paid by insurance. Referring to the folder and being able to advise the hospital of the claim date, payment date and amount paid resolved the issue quickly.

Provider	Provided	Date	Claim Amt	Sent	Date/Amt Pd
Doctor	Ofc Call	11/2	85.00	11/15	11/30-85.00
Lab	Blood Test	11/8	118.00	11/30	

At this point, the main issue is "keep it simple". My suggested method is a twenty-nine cent school folder, with pockets front and back. All the bills go into the middle as they are received. When I got the chance, I made out a claim form, copied the form and all the bills going with it, and mailed the originals. I placed the copies in the front pocket and entered the information in the log. When I received notification that insurance had paid that claim or when I received a check for medication, I noted the payment on the log and the notification letter and copies were moved to the back pocket with the payment statement.

In addition to helping me know where we were financially, if payment of a bill was questioned, I knew whether a claim had been filed and if it had shown paid. I could easily identify unpaid claims and question the insurance company or Veterans Administration office as to why payment was delayed.

In the event you must do any traveling for treatment, try to do it all on credit cards. Charge plane tickets, car rentals, hotels, even meals when possible. Some of this may be reimbursed by insurance, some by your local cancer society. And, the information is invaluable when filing taxes for those expenses that no one reimbursed. Expense information is also necessary if you file for any Veteran Administration benefits, Social Security benefits or in the event you end up filing a law suit based upon the cause of cancer.

If your local pharmacy honors charge cards or will set up an account for your prescriptions, this can make life a lot easier. Not only can other people pick up the prescriptions if you have listed them as potential couriers, but billings come once a month and can be paid with proceeds from the insurance medication claim checks.

In Walt's case we billed between five hundred and a thousand dollars in drugs during our seven weeks home from Seattle. As we had no income at the time, this was money we could not afford to spend out of pocket. I could bill the insurance company from the prescription billings once a week and pay the drug store as the claims were settled.

Disability Claims
Insurance/Social Security/V.A.

This is another of those practical issues that truly need to be handled at a time when all you want to do is cry, scream, and rage at the unfairness of life or simply spend one hundred percent of your time with your loved one.

With the exception of some insurance companies, most agencies base their waiting periods and payment periods on the date the claim was filed, not the date the disability started or income stopped. So if you go to

Social Security only when you realize that your loved one's sick pay or other disability pay ended, you will have to wait five months more before payments begin.

Whether you are filing for Social Security disability, service related disability for a veteran, non-service related disability for a veteran or for insurance disability, be prepared to fill out more forms than you ever care to think about seeing. In many instances, agencies will require documentation to evaluate your level of need. This may be anything from the DD214 military form to your most recent bank statements. If you have a friend or family member who can help you track down paperwork, make copies of completed forms or deliver the unending stream of forms to the agencies, take advantage of that help.

13

Practical Considerations of Life and Death

-NOVEMBER 8TH -

Thank God for small towns and caring nurses. Got a call this morning that the admitting doctor in the emergency room left an order for life support system use, something Walt emphatically does not want, and he's so sedated he's not even coherent. I managed to get the order reversed.

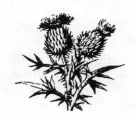

N ot very many of us recognize the importance of a Power of Attorney and few of us have one. After my experience with Walt, when I remarried recently, my husband and I discussed the value of the Power of Attorney and of wills. Still, the only reason we currently have both is that he took a consulting job that required traveling out of the country several times a year. That fact made us aware that either of us could have an accident while the other was an ocean away. More practically, without his power of attorney I would have been unable to deposit our joint IRS refund; unable to pick up his checks from the contracting firm; unable to act on the paperwork necessary to complete the refinancing of the house, a process which had been started before he left and had to be completed before his scheduled return.

With a terminal illness, the importance of a Power of Attorney may be a matter of life or death. Some very real examples follow: The patient is heavily sedated and they need to do surgery or begin treatment; for whatever reason, the patient begins hallucinating whether due to medication, lack of sleep or tumor location; the patient is on morphine; the patient is in a coma. You must have the authority to make decisions for the patient in these circumstances.

In some hospitals, it is standard procedure to initiate artificial life support systems unless the patient has stated otherwise. Depending upon your feelings about artificial life support, this could be a critical issue if your loved one is admitted and is not capable of requesting the waiver or is simply not aware of this fact. It almost happened to us.

From a practical, day-to-day standpoint, some insurance companies will not accept medical claim forms unless signed by the insured employee. In other words, the spouse's signature is not considered valid. This was true of Walt's insurance company. Do you, along with everything else, want to continue shoving insurance forms in front of your spouse, especially if he/she has suddenly become ultra-concerned about the expense of the disease?

Depending on how your checking accounts are set up and the policies of your bank, you may not be able to deposit pay checks and/or insurance checks made out to your loved one. The employer may not be willing to release sick-leave or disability checks to you.

If you don't have a Power of Attorney, as we did not, there is no good time to introduce this form, even though it can become a critical document. We both assigned Power of Attorney when the issue of my picking up his paycheck arose.

When Walt was admitted to the hospital the last time, the doctor on duty that night had stipulated artificial life support to be used if Walt ceased breathing. Walt was then on four liters of oxygen per minute. I knew he was definitely against artificial life support; however, because he was so medicated, he was not asked. With the Power of Attorney, I was able to reverse the doctor's instructions.

After Walt was on morphine, the doctor needed my permission to do a final lung tap. The Power of Attorney allowed me to check Walt out of the hospital for his final return home.

A copy of the format we used for Power of Attorney is included in the Appendices.

Wills

It is my heartfelt hope that you already have wills prepared as you are reading this. We did not—one of the many things we had never gotten around to—and this was one of the more difficult practical things we had to deal with. One minute you agree that "We're going to beat this thing," and the next you say "But please sign this will." In our case, the issue was made somewhat easier by our pastor who was aware of all the circumstances of our situation.

We were not wealthy and so could use the basic format of the sample shown in the Appendices and pretty much fill in the blanks. Since I had a computer and word processing program, completing the will was relatively simple from a mechanical standpoint. Walt and I made out our wills at the same time. None the less, doing so in his hospital room was far from ideal. Walt's will was signed and witnessed just three and a half days before his death. One of the witnesses was the head floor nurse, as suggested by Pastor George in the event there was any question of Walt's mental competence at that stage of his illness.

You need to be aware that without a will the State often determines settlement of the estate and if there are children or step-children involved, the widow may end up with as little as twenty-five percent of the assets; to say nothing of dealing with frozen bank accounts, sealed safety deposit boxes and a twelve month waiting period while the estate sits in probate court and no one can touch anything or sell anything. I know very few people who feel that a court could best determine where the individual would like their assets to go.

Wills and requirements vary from state to state. After looking at the sample provided in the Appendices (used in the states of Alaska and Florida), your best source is a local attorney or stationary store. They should carry the standard will form used in your area.

If your situation is anything other than very simple, it is probably best to have the will reviewed by an attorney. The money spent to have an attorney review or draw up your wills could save you thousands of dollars and a lot of trouble in the future. Challenges to the will by parents, siblings, former spouses, stepchildren or illegitimate children can be devastating at a time when you are trying to put your life together.

Living Wills

A Living Will simply states that you want the right to die with dignity. It releases your physician from the responsibility of administering artificial life support to prolong the wait for iminent death. The Living Will is not legally recognized in all states at this time, although more and more states are adopting such an alternative.

The sample included in the Appendices conforms to Washington state laws. Check with your local attorney or physician to see if your state recognizes the Living Will. If so, stationery stores should carry the appropriate forms, similar to the one shown in the appendices.

Complete three or four originals of this document. One should be given to your physician, a copy kept with your will, one given to a close friend and one kept at your house. It's a good idea to keep originals of the Living Will, the Power of Attorney, and your Wills in a safety deposit box with other important papers. The Living Will should be easy to locate, as it could be needed in an emergency situation. For example if you are in an automobile accident away from home your personal physician would not be treating you in this situation and the unknown attending physician would need to be provided a copy of the Living Will. If copies have been made and distributed, it will be easier to verify that you do have such a document and get a copy when needed.

The Practical Matters of Death

As with the illness, there are practical considerations when death occurs. There are numerous books available on dealing with death and I am not going to reiterate information you can find elsewhere. I am however, going to include another checklist.

1. Request an autopsy. This is particularly important if there is any reason to suspect the loved one's cancer was caused by an outside factor, such as asbestos or Agent Orange. An autopsy may be the only thing that will assure you of veteran benefits for the widow. An autopsy may be necessary to verify in-process disability claims or other insurance benefits. Be sure the hospice or home health care nurse and the coroner understand that you want an autopsy done.

2. Request at least a dozen copies of the Death Certificate. You will be amazed at the number of people who require this document: every life insurance company the loved one had a policy with; the Veterans Administration; the group health carrier, if coverage included a small life

policy; the mortgage department at the bank; the employer and the administrator of any pension, profit-sharing, or retirement plans; and the social security office.

3. Check on available burial benefits. We were eligible for benefits from Social Security and from the Veterans Administration. In addition, the State of Alaska Veterans Affairs division provided burial benefits for resident veterans. There may also be benefits available from fraternal organizations your loved one belonged to.

14
The Final Days

NOVEMBER 17TH -

Walt's day nurse indicates we're near the end; his night nurse says he'll see Christmas. I don't see how he can make it through tonight, his breathing is so labored and the morphine has him so zonked.

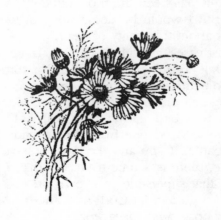

"Ignore it, and maybe it'll go away". I tried to do that with Walt's battle with cancer. Shelly tried to do it as Dave's condition worsened. Mom tried the same philosophy when Dad was in Bartlett Hospital his last few days. And I tried to do it with this book. Fortunately I have friends and mentors who forced me to once again deal with reality.

A terminal illness is exactly what is says. Final. An ending. This has been the most difficult part of the book to write. But I would be doing none of us a favor if we didn't talk about the reality of death.

In most cases, as with Dad, Walt, Dave, John, the end is a blessing. Terminal cancer is uncomfortable, unpleasant and sometimes unbearable. An end may be what you are hoping and praying for.

Don't feel bad. Don't feel guilty. In truth, death releases your loved one from the constant pain and the constant battle. If you and the doctors have done all that is possible, there is a time to accept that a Higher Being has plans that supersede your own dreams of the future. Time to "Let go and let God" as Catherine Marshall counsels in her book *Something More*.

I said I wanted to be there for you, that I wanted this book to take the place of a phone call or kitchen chat.

Let me tell you about my experiences, the days before and the days after. Let me open my journal for your review.

> WEDNESDAY, NOVEMBER 6
> *...Walt has been like a zombie all day. Respiration sounded so bad I called Judy. We took Walt to the hospital tonight so they can level out the medication there. ...I, of course, cry a lot. It's so frustrating. But it will be so nice for both of us to get a couple of day's rest and then have him back home and coherent.*

I was near the breaking point. We had been on a roller coaster of pain, medication, little if any sleep for either of us. When we took Walt to the emergency room, it was to be for two days of supervised medication experimenting. The goal was to find a combination that would assure he was not in pain and still allow him to function.

> THURSDAY, NOVEMBER 7
> *...Back to the hospital at 6:00, Walt slept most of the time I was there. I am really beginning to fear that things aren't working and that all we have is a short period of time. I knew this was a strong possibility, but hadn't really accepted it. My constant prayer is that if he has to go, he won't have to suffer.*

I spent hours in tears that night. While I am not a psychic nor do I believe in hearing voices, I felt that Someone had said to me, "Get ready. Walt isn't going to see Thanksgiving." That night I faced the very real possibility that I would lose my husband. Finally admitting that fact allowed me to grieve for myself, for Walt, for his kids, for our friends. It also allowed me to let go of Walt. To this point, I had selfishly wanted him with me always, regardless. I began to realize that having him with me in pain, frustrated by his own dependence on others, was not what either of us wanted.

Hospice and Shanti believe that the cancer patient is aware of this subconscious holding on by the loved one. This awareness may cause a great deal of anxiety, because the loved one is ready to die and has recognized that the only way this is going to get better is when it's over. One of the biggest favors you can do your loved one is to face this reality yourself and find a way to deal with it.

Walt and I never talked about that night; Walt rarely saw me cry. But I think Walt knew somehow that I had come to terms with the reality of our situation. That freed him to come to terms with it himself.

SUNDAY, NOVEMBER 10
...Walt is so much better. Breathing well and absolutely no confusion. Visits from Favors, Heusslers, family. Tucked Walt in and headed home about 11:00. ...He seems chilled and has sniffles. A cold is the last thing he needs right now.

WEDNESDAY, NOVEMBER 13
Things look so good today I can hardly believe it. Walt is feeling great. We gave him a shower and they started the slow drip chemotherapy. As soon as that's done, three days I think, Walt can come home!   ...Dr. Frank talked with Dr. C and both seem pleased with Walt's progress. ...

THURSDAY, NOVEMBER 14
Walt took a walk around the halls and we visited briefly with Annie who is at the end of the hall. He went almost half an hour without the oxygen, just the portable IV. Dr. Frank was quite pleased and talked about gradually reducing the oxygen level in an effort to get him off oxygen in the not too distant future.

Coming to terms with the reality obviously doesn't preclude hoping you're wrong. Once they started leveling out the medications, we had some super days, even though Walt was still in the hospital for the chemotherapy treatments. We laughed, talked about what we were going to do in the spring and planned long relaxing weekends on the boat.

It was a good time, time we needed together to pretend that everything was going to be all right, real soon.

FRIDAY, NOVEMBER 15
I think we need to eliminate Fridays for Walt. He had another rough day. Chest pains started about 7:00 or 8:00 am. By the time I got to the hospital they had started morphine. He was in agonizing pain until 3:30 and they finally loaded him with morphine. He's better this evening and did a good job on dinner.

SUNDAY, NOVEMBER 17
Walt called me at 9:15 am—couldn't sleep and wanted to come home today! They completed the slow drip chemo at 8:00 and he doesn't understand why he has to stay a minute longer. Dr. Frank called at 10:00 for permission to do thorentecis. Walt's day nurse indicates we're near the end; his night nurse says he'll see Christmas. I don't see how he can make it through tonight, his breathing is so labored and the morphine has him semi-zonked.

I didn't even undress that night when I went to bed. I was sure I would receive a call in the middle of the night, a summons to the hospital.

It was the next day that Walt actually came home. I had been on the telephone all evening Sunday, trying to locate a private duty nurse, someone who could come out to the house and be with me when I brought Walt home. The tumor had broken through the lung wall and invaded the entire lung area, possibly the brain. Dr. Frank had prescribed morphine given intravenously. This was one of those times where I said "I can't do this." I knew that an injection, given wrongly, could kill Walt almost instantly and I couldn't take that responsibility. Unfortunately there are very few private duty nurses in a small town and I could find none available on short notice.

When I arrived at the hospital Monday morning, Walt had his end of the hall in a minor uproar. He had been up since six-thirty, was dressed, had all his belongings in his suitcase and was ready to go home. The nurses were at their wit's end, trying to keep him from going down to the lobby to wait for me.

By nine-thirty, the room was crowded and had the appearance of a high level staff meeting. That's exactly what it was. Walt, the doctor, the hospice nurse, the floor nurse, my mother and I were all trying to figure out the mechanics of getting Walt home and trying to explain to him why we needed a nurse there without causing him unnecessary concern. Into the middle of this walked Ellen, a surgical nurse at the hospital and a dear friend of ours.

Much like a child, Walt finally said that he'd stay another day if he really had to, but reminded me that "you promised I could come home as soon as I finished my chemo."

Ellen assessed the situation immediately. She said, "Walt, if you want to go home, I'll come over and stay tonight."

I immediately asked the doctor to sign the release papers and we took Walt home.

Although we didn't verbalize it at the time, I knew and Walt knew that we had reached the end and that end was not going to be in a hospital. It was going to be in his own home. Mom made the necessary phone calls, tracking down his girls, while the hospice nurse helped me get Walt settled and left to make the necessary arrangements. In the event of an expected home death, many of the details of death normally handled by hospital staff must be done by the family or home nursing team. Mary alerted the State Troopers and the mortuary to the possibility of Walt's death.

Ellen came over that evening. It was clear that it was only a matter of time. The problem with cancer is that time can be hours or days or weeks. This is part of what is so extremely painful, knowing there is nothing more to be done, that the battle can't be won, and yet your loved one is still a prisoner of pain. All you can do is wait. And hope. And pray. And allow yourself to want it to be over, admit to the desire and need for peace and release for both of you.

Several hours after she arrived, Ellen told me that if Walt made it through the night, he would have to go back to the hospital in the morning. There was no way we could care for his needs at home. She assured me that he wouldn't know where he was, he was too heavily sedated and would have to remain that way. I remember my response. "If we can't beat this thing, if he has to die, I hope he dies here tonight, surrounded by our friends."

Walt died at three o'clock the following morning with Ellen by his side.

15

The Emotions
of Death

-NOVEMBER 20TH -

Feeling basically numb...

Call from the doctor—he got back into town this morning and is taking Walt's death pretty hard also. ...I leak a lot (Chuck's term) and feel pretty fragmented.

Mom and Carol over for several hours, Ellen stopped for coffee, several calls, Deb still staying here. So many caring people... although at times I feel smothered and over-protected.

Many of the emotions at the death of a loved one are the same emotions felt at the time of diagnosis and throughout the illness. Understanding and accepting them now is as critical as it was when you were coping with cancer. Although the circumstances have changed, many of the rules have not. Most of the suggestions are still valid. What you feel is okay. You don't have to meet anyone else's conception of right and wrong, should and ought. You can still exercise the option of ignoring sentences containing these two words, unless they deal with accomplishing a practical task that must be done.

Obviously denial is no longer an option. If denial has been your primary coping method, the death may be much harder to accept and adjust to. Denial eliminates the ability to grieve prior to the actual death.

You may be angry. I was at times. And why not? After all your efforts and hard work, your loved one is gone and you are left behind, alone, abandoned, to figure out how to continue living, how to handle daily details, how to put your life back together. It isn't fair. And it isn't easy. But it can be done.

You may experience resentment. Regardless of the fact that all you want to do is crawl under a rock, there are still a lot of details that have to be handled almost immediately: Write an obituary with a friend's help. Return the hospital equipment. Make decisions on a memorial service or funeral. Answer questions from the coroner or mortuary. And there is still paperwork to do. Of course you're going to resent these intrusions into your grief. They aren't going to go away, so allow yourself to resent them and then take care of what you can.

In my case I used all these tasks and duties to keep myself busy and insulate myself from some portion of the grief. Oh I cried a lot, but didn't allow myself time to worry or wail. You may well do the same thing. However, don't be surprised when the day of reckoning arrives. It may be a week, it may be a month, it may be a year or more; but one day it will become very clear just exactly what has happened and what that means to you.

On that day of reckoning, your world crumbles around your ears and you wonder if you can go on, why you should have to go on—alone. The pain is a physical ache and you began to understand that there is reality to the term heartbreak. When that occurs, I sincerely hope you will allow yourself the time, the freedom and the compassion to fall apart and allow the fears and anger to flow out of you, along with the tears. This is the moment that marks the beginning of recovery and, once it occurs, you'll be better able to pick up the pieces and go on.

You may want to check with American Cancer Society, your hospice team, the Visiting Nurse's Association or your church to see if there are support groups in your area for dealing with grief and loss. Society has finally recognized that each and every one of us must deal with loss at some point in life. Just as coping with the illness is easier when one talks with others in the same situation, so dealing with your loss is easier when you are in contact with others who can appreciate what you're going through, what you have gone through and what you are currently facing.

There may be any number of people who are ready and willing to offer advice. The rule for accepting advice now is the same as it was during your loved one's illness: If a statement begins with "should" or "ought" you have no obligation to listen to or implement the suggestion. Each and every one of us must deal with grief in our own way and each and every one of us has our own timetable for acceptance and renewal. Accept the fact that what you're feeling this week is probably not what you will be feeling next week or next month. This is not the time to make major decisions about changing jobs, changing careers or changing residence if you have the option of maintaining the status quo for six months or so.

Allow yourself time to grieve and give yourself permission to grieve in your own way. You have been through a situation that is unlike any that most of your friends and relatives have experienced, even if they have lost a loved one. My mother and I dealt with our grief in different ways and on different timetables. Shelly and I dealt with our grief in different ways and on different timetables. There is no right or wrong, there is only what is right for you.

After the Fact

My first thought, when Ellen told me Walt had died was "Thank God".

I can admit that now. It is a valid and sincere reaction to the end of pain and frustration for your loved one and for you.

A friend in Florida took care of his father during a year-long battle with cancer. Bob gave up a successful business to care for his father twenty-four hours a day, providing the nursing care that his father needed and that Bob felt only he could provide. One day, when we were talking about this book, we discussed the inclusion of death. That day Bob admitted to me:

"Maybe it's a terrible thing, but I can still remember one of the first thoughts I had as I held Dad in my arms after he died, 'I'm free.' Does that make me a terrible person?"

Absolutely not! You have poured heart and soul, energy and time, love and compassion into the battle with cancer. Our reactions, such as "Thank God, it's over", "I'm free", "It's finally ended" are as normal a response to the end of the battle with cancer as they would be coming from a soldier at the end of a war.

In many cases we have done a great deal of grieving throughout the process of nursing our loved ones. You may have been living for days or weeks with the knowledge that there was only one resolution to the battle so the relief you feel when there is no more to be done, no more pain to be endured, no more frustration to be borne, is probably one of the first positive emotions you've had for some time. And it's okay.

And believe it or not, one day the sun will look a little brighter, you'll discover a higher level of energy and you will sincerely smile and laugh at someone or something. You'll find a rekindling of old interests or discover a new interest that truly intrigues you. You'll want to go to a social event, instead of forcing yourself to go. And you will always be aware of life's priorities and the importance of taking risks and enjoying every day, every event, every experience. This advantage is reserved for those of us who have been there.

Bibliography

Garfield, Charles A. "The Impact of Death on the Health-Care Professional." Shanti Project article, 1977.

LeGette, Bernard. *LeGette's Calorie Encyclopedia*. Warner Books, 1983.

Marshall, Catherine. *Something More*. Avon Books, 1974.

Muir, John D. *Why Die At Home*. Muir Publishing, 1977.

Prather, Hugh. *I Touch the Earth, The Earth Touches Me*. Doubleday & Co, 1972.

——————. *Notes To Myself*. Real People Press, 1970.

Vietnam Veterans of America. *Viet Vet Survival Guide*. 1st Edition. Bantam, 1985.

Appendix A
First Week Checklist

1. Buy a 3"x 5" or 5" x 8" three hole notebook.
   Start logging doctors visits; expenses; recommended agencies for assistance, etc..

2. Call American Cancer Society.
   (See Appendix B for numbers)

3. Charge everything.

4. Start an expense folder..

5. Contact your insurance company(s).

6. Call Social Security disability office.

7. Contact the Veterans Administration.

8. Contact any local, state or federal agencies listed under Social Services who may be able to help you.

9. Contact a friend with the ability to copy forms and claims for you.

Appendix B
Check List
for Coming Home

1. Home health care requirements established

2. Prescriptions, medications, especially for pain

3. Equipment, i.e. hospital bed, wheel chair, shower chair, commode, bedpan or urinal, walker, crutches.

4. Extra sheets and bedding

5. Several flat flannel sheets

6. Egg crate mattress—for as many of the beds as the patient may opt to use (these are often part of what you'll bring home from the hospital).

7. Extra nightgowns or nightshirts if patient uses them.

8. Drinking straws that bend

9. Extra pillows

10. Tissues

11. Socks & non-skid slippers

12. Anything your spouse was using in the hospital that you will also need at home and that you've already paid for.

13. Full supply of groceries

14. Med charts from home health care unit

15. You may want to consider an in-house monitor like they make for nurseries if your house is large or on two levels. This allows you to monitor the patient at all times and still allows you to move freely around the house, garage, basement and yard.

Appendix C
Medical Abbreviations

Prescriptions are generally written in medical language. Since it is quite possible you may not remember the doctor's verbal instructions when he gives you a prescription, the list below explains the medical shorthand found on many prescriptions.

a.	Before
a.c.	Before food or meals
ad lib	To the amount desired
b.i.d., b.d.	Two times a day
b.i.n., b.n.	Two times a night
b.m.r.	Basal metabolism rate
b.p.	Blood pressure
c., c.	With
e.g.	For example
ext.	Extract
fl.	Fluid
gtt(s).	A drop, drops

h.s.	At bedtime
I.M.	Intramuscular
I.V.	Intravenous
noct.	At night
NPO	Nothing by mouth
p.o.	Give orally
p.r.n.	As needed
q.d.	Every day
q.i.d.	Four times a day
q.o.d.	Every other day
Sx	Symptoms
t.i.d.	Three times a day
Tx	Treatments
MS, OMS	Morphine solution

Appendix D
Med Chart

Date				
Medication				
Dose				
Time Taken				
By Whom				
Instructions				
Comments				

Appendix E
Organizations
That Help

American Cancer Society, Inc

1599 Clifton Road N.E.
Atlanta GA 30329
(404) 320-3333

The American Cancer Society offers education, patient services and rehabilitation, service programs for patients and families, counseling, community health service referrals, equipment loans, transportation and is particularly helpful in instances where you must travel to another location to receive the necessary treatment or care.

The American Cancer Society has a nation-wide toll free number that will automatically route calls to the nearest ACS office. Call 1-800-ACS-2345 (1-800-227-2345) and your call will reach the nearest office in your area. The State chapters are listed on the following pages.

Alabama Division, Inc.
402 Office Park Dr., Suite 300
Birmingham AL 35223
(205) 879-2242

Alaska Division, Inc.
406 W. Fireweed La. Suite 204
Anchorage AK 99503
(907) 227-8696

Arizona Division, Inc.
2929 E. Thomas Rd.
Phoenix AZ 85016
(601) 224-0524

Arkansas Division, Inc.
901 N. University
Little Rock AR 72207
(501) 664-3480

California Division, Inc.
1710 Webster St.
P.O. Box 2061
Oakland CA 94612
(415) 893-7900

Colorado Division, Inc.
2255 South Oneida
P.O. Box 24669
Denver CO 80224
(303) 748-2030

Connecticut Division, Inc.
Barnes Park South
14 Village Lane
Wallingford CT 06492
(203) 265-7161

Delaware Division, Inc.
1708 Lovering Avenue
Suite 202
Wilmington DE 19806
(302) 654-5267

District of Columbia Division
1825 Connecticut Ave, NW
Suite 315
Washington DC 20009
(202) 483-2600

Florida Division, Inc.
1001 So. MacDill Avenue
Tampa FL 33629
(813) 253-0541

Georgia Division, Inc.
46 Fifth Street NE
Atlanta GA 30308
(404) 892-0026

Hawaii/Pacific Division, Inc.
Community Services Center
200 No. Vineyard Blvd.
Honolulu HI 96817
(808) 531-1662

Idaho Division, Inc.
2676 Vista Avenue
P.O. Box 5386
Boise ID 83705
(208) 343-4609

Illinois Division, Inc.
77 E. Monroe
Chicago IL 60603
(312) 641-6150

Indiana Division, Inc.
8730 Commercial Park Place
Indianapolis IN 46268
(317) 872-4432

Iowa Division, Inc.
8364 Hickman Road, Suite D
Des Moines IA 50322
(515) 253-0147

Kansas Division, Inc.
1315 S.W. Arrowhead Road
Topeka KS 66604
(913 273-4114

Kentucky Division, Inc.
701 W. Muhammad Ali Blvd.
P.O. Box 1807
Louisville KY 40201-1807
(502) 584-6782

Louisiana Division, Inc.
Fidelity Homestead Bldg
837 Gravier St., Suite 700
New Orleans LA 70112-1509
(504 523-4188

Maine Division, Inc.
52 Federal St.
Brunswick ME 04011
(207) 729-3339

Maryland Division, Inc.
8219 Town Center Dr.
White Marsh MD 21162-0082
(301) 529-7272

Massachusetts Division, Inc.
247 Commonwealth Ave.
Boston MA 02116
(617) 267-2650

Michigan Division, Inc.
1205 E. Saginaw St.
Lansing MI 48906
(517) 371-2920

Minnesota Division, Inc.
3316 W. 66th St.
Minneapolis MN 55435
(612) 925-2772

Mississippi Division, Inc.
1380 Livingston La.
Lakeover Office Park
Jackson MS 39213
(601) 362-8874

Missouri Division, Inc.
3322 American Avenue
Jefferson City MO 65102
(314) 893-4800

Montana Division, Inc.
313 N. 32nd St., Suite #1
Billings MT 59101
(406) 252-7111

Nebraska Division, Inc.
8502 W. Center Rd.
Omaha NE 68124-5255
(402) 393-5800

Nevada Division, Inc.
1325 E. Harmon
Las Vegas NV 89119
(702) 798-6857

New Hampshire Division, Inc.
360 Route 101, Unit 501
Bedford NH 03102-6800
(603) 472-8899

New Jersey Division, Inc.
2600 Route 1, CNN 2201
North Brunswick NJ 08902
(201) 297-8000

New Mexico Division, Inc.
5800 Lomas Blvd, NE
Albuquerque NM 87110
(505) 262-2336

New York State Division, Inc.
6725 Lyons Street
P.O. Box 7
East Syracuse NY 13057
(315) 437-7025

Long Island Division, Inc.
145 Pidgeon Hill Rd.
Huntington Station NY 11746
(516) 385-9100

New York City Division, Inc.
19 W 56th St.
New York NY 10019
(212) 586-8700

Queens Division, Inc.
112-25 Queens Blvd
Forest Hills NY 11375
(718) 263-2224

Westchester Division, Inc.
30 Glenn St.
White Plains NY 11375
(914) 949-4800

North Carolina Division, Inc.
11 South Boylan Avenue, #221
Raleigh NC 27603
(919) 834-8463

North Dakota Division, Inc.
123 Roberts St.
P.O. Box 426
Fargo ND 58107

Ohio Division, Inc.
5555 Frantz Road
Dublin OH 43017
(614) 889-9565

Oklahoma Division, Inc.
3000 United Founders Blvd.,
Suite 136
Oklahoma City OK 73112
(405) 843-9888

Oregon Division, Inc.
0330 SW Curry
Portland Oregon 97201
(503) 295-6422

Pennsylvania Division, Inc.
P.O. Box 897
Route 422 & Sipe Avenue
Hershey PA 17033-0897
(717) 533-6144

Philadelphia Division, Inc.
1325 Chestnut St.
Philadelphia PA 19102
(215) 665-2900

Puerto Rico Division, Inc.
Calle Alverio #577
Esquina Sargento Medina
Hato Rey, PR 00918
(809) 764-2295

Rhode Island Division, Inc.
400 Main St.
Pawtucket RI 02860
(401) 722-8480

South Carolina Division, Inc.
128 Stonemark Lane
Columbia SC 29210
(803) 750-1693

South Dakota Division, Inc.
4101 Carnegie Place
Sioux Falls SD 57106-8277
(605) 361-8277

Tennessee Division, Inc.
1315 Eighth Avenue S.
Nashville TN 37203
(615) 255-1227

Texas Division, Inc.
2433 Ridgepoint Drive
Austin TX 78754
(512) 928-2262

Utah Division, Inc.
610 E. South Temple
Salt Lake City UT 84102
(801) 322-0431

Vermont Division, Inc.
13 Loomis St., Drawer C
P.O. Box 1452
Montpelier VT 05601-1452
(802) 223-2348

Virginia Division, Inc.
4240 Park Place Court
Glen Allen VA 23060
(804) 270-0142

Washington Division, Inc.
2120 First Avenue No.
Seattle WA 98109-1140
(206) 283-1152

West Virginia Division, Inc.
2428 Kanawha Blvd. E.
Charleston WV 25311
(304) 344-3611

Wisconsin Division, Inc.
615 No Sherman Ave
Madison WI 53704
(608) 249-0487

Wyoming Division, Inc.
2222 House Avenue
Cheyenne WY 82001
(307) 638-3331

Hospice

1901 North Ft. Myer Drive
Arlington VA 22209
(703) 243-5900

The hospice organization is made up of health professionals and volunteers and provides practical, medical and emotional support for the cancer patient, the caregiver and the family. Services provided by hospice are paid for by insurance or through the program itself; the family usually never sees an invoice for services provided.

The following list indicates the state hospice associations and their phone numbers to help you in locating hospice assistance in your area.

Alabama Hospice Organization
912 River Haven Circle
Hoover AL 35244
(205) 733-0166

Hospice of Anchorage
3605 Artic Blvd, #555
Anchorage AK 99503
(907) 561-5322

Arizona Hospice Organization
East Valley Hospice
1450 S. Dobson, Suite B-322
Mesa AZ 85202
(602) 835-0711

Arkansas State Hospice
1501 N University, Suite 400
Little Rock AR 72207
(501) 664-7870

Hospice of the Ozarks
21 Medical Plaza
Mountain Home AR 72653
(501) 425-2797

California State Hospice
P.O. Box 1186
Torrance CA 90510
(213) 534-5600

Colorado State Hospice
P.O. Box 2270
Evergreen CO 80439
(303) 674-6400

Hospice Council of
Connecticut
205 West Main St.
New Britain CT 096052
(203) 224-7131

Hospice Council of
Connecticut
60 Lorraine St.
Hartford CT 06105
(203) 233-2222

Delaware Hospice, Inc.
3519 Silverside Rd., Suite 100
Rigdely Bldg
Wilmington DE 19810
(302) 478-5707

Metropolitan Hospice Council
Hospice Care of the DC
1749 St. Matthews Ct., NW
Washington DC 20036
(202) 347-1700

Florida Hospices, Inc.
P.O. Box 560965
Rockledge FL 32956
(407) 636-2211

Georgia Hospice Organization
Hospice of Athens
2092 Prince Avenue
Athens GA 30606
(404) 548-8923

Hawaii State Hospice Network
St. Francis Medical Center
24 Puiwa Road
Honolulu HI 96817
(808) 537-6011

Idaho Hospice Organization
Hospice of North Idaho
2003 Lincoln Way
Coeur d'Alene ID 83814
(208) 667-4537

Illinois State Hospice
Organization
Hospice of the North Shore
P.O. Box 398
Wilmette IL 60091
(312) 866-4601

Illinois State Hospice
Organization
305 S Illinois St., Suite 100
Belleville IL 62220
(618) 235-7755

Indiana Assoc. of Hospices
St. Vincent Hospice
P.O. Box 80160
Indianapolis IN 46280
(317) 874-4696

Iowa Hospice Organization
Cedar Valley Hospice
200 E. Ridgeway, Suite 200
Waterloo IA 50702
(319) 292-1450

Iowa Hospice Organization
8364 Hickman Rd., Suite D
Des Moines IA 50322
(515) 253-0875

Kansas State Hospice
Organization
Phillips County Area Hospice
Box 607
Phillipsburg KS 67661
(913) 543-5226, ext 250

Kentucky Assoc. of Hospices
Lourdes Hospice
1530 Lone Oak Rd.
Paducah KY 42002
(502) 444-2262

Louisiana Hospice
Organization
Schumpert Medical Center 335
Margaret Place
Shreveport LA 71120
(318) 227-4605

Maine Hospice Council
11 Parkwood Drive
Augusta ME 04330
(27) 622-7566

Hospice Network of Maryland
Hospice of P G County
96 Harry Truman Dr.
Largo MD 20772
(301) 499-0550

Hospice Network of Maryland
5820 S. Western Blvd
Suite 100-A
Baltimore MD 21227
(301) 242-1975

Hospice Care at Southwood
Community Hospital
111 Dedham St.
Norfolk MA 02056
(508) 668-0385

Michigan Hospice Organization
233 E. Fulton
Suite 210
Grand Rapids MI 49503
(616) 454-1426

Minnesota Hospice
Organization
Hospice of Healtheast
69 W. Exchange St.
St. Paul MN 55102
(612) 291-3544

Minnesota Hospice
Organization
Riverside Medical Center
25th and Riverside
Minneapolis MN 55454
(612) 337-4217

Mississippi
Gulf Coast Comm. Hospice
545 - 16th St, #36
Gulfport MS 39507
(601) 896-7483

Missouri Hospice Organization
9414 Pine Avenue
St. Louis MO 63144
(314) 962-9115

Montana Hospice Organization
Mountain West HH & Hospice
500 No. Higgins, Suite 201
Missoula MT 59802
(406) 728-8848

Nebraska Hospice Org.
Home Health
Beatrice Community Hospital
1201 So. Ninth
Beatrice NE 68310
(402) 223-2366

Nevada
Nathan Adelson Hospice
4141 S. Swenson St.
Las Vegas NV 89119
(702) 733-0320

New Hampshire
Home Health & Hospice Care
22 Prospect St.
Nashua NH 03060
(603) 882-2941

New Jersey Hospice
Organization
Medical Center Hospice
1 Riverview Plaza
Redbank NJ 07701
(201) 530-2382

New Jersey Hospice
Organization
Center for Health Affairs
760 Alexander Rd., CN-1
Princeton NJ 08540
(609) 275-4125

New Mexico Association for
Home Care
1339 Cerrillus Rd., Suite 6
Sante Fe NM 87501
(505) 982-9962

Mesilla Valley Hospice
225 E. Idaho, Suite 23
Las Cruces NM 88005
(505) 523-4700

New York State Hospice
Association
Hospice Care Inc.
409 Mandeville St.
Utica NY 13502

New York State Hospice
Association
468 Rosedale Avenue
White Plains NY 10605
(914) 946-7699

Hospice of North Carolina
Hospice of Wake County
1307 Glenwood Avenue
Raleigh NC 27605
(919) 833-9521

Hospice of North Carolina
1046 Washington St.
Raleigh NC 27605
(919) 829-9588

North Dakota Hospice
Organization
United Hospice
1133 S. Columbia Rd.
Grand Forks ND 58201
(701) 780-5258

Ohio Hospice Organization
3137 W. Broad St.
Columbus OH 43204
(614) 274-9513

Oklahoma Hospice
Organization
Eastern Oklahoma Hospice
2012 A West Okmulgee
Muskogee OK 74401
(918) 683-1192

Oregon Hospice Association
P.O. Box 10796
Portland OR 97210
(503) 228-2104

Pennsylvania Hospice
Network
Hospice Care, Inc.
P.O. Box 1316,
55 Highland Ave
Washington PA 15301
(412) 627-8118

Puerto Rico
Hospicio La Providencia
P.O. Box 10447
Ponce PR 00732
(809) 843-2364

Hospice Care of Rhode Island
345 Blackstone Blvd
Providence RI 02906
(401) 272-4900

Hospice of South Carolina
Hospice of Anderson
800 N. Fant St.
Anderson SC 29501
(803) 662-2978

Hospice of South Carolina
1807 Marsh Avenue
Florence SC 29501
(803) 662-2978

Tennessee State Hospice
Organization
Hospice of Murfreesboro
310 No. University
Murfreesboro TN 37130

Texas Hospice Organization
1600 Heather Glen Ct.
Richardson TX 75081
(214) 783-1457

Utah Hospice Organization
Hospice of IHC Home Care
1875 S. State T500
Orem UT 85048
(801) 225-0584

Hospice Council of Vermont
Hospice of Lamoile
RR 1, Box 2300
Stowe VT 05672
(802) 253-8572

Hospice Council of Vermont
52 State St.
Montpelier VT 05602
(802) 229-9579

Virginia Association
for Hospices
Hospice of Williamsburg
P.O. Box 568
Williamsburg VA 23185
(804) 253-1220

Hospice Council
of West Virginia
Hospice of Huntington
P.O. Box 464
Huntington WV 25701
(304) 529-4217

Virginia Association
for Hospices
7814 Carousel Ln, Suite 300
Richmond VA 23229
(804) 346-0862

Wisconsin Hospice
Organization
7 No. Pinckney, Suite 119
Madison WI 53703
(608)257-2611

Washington Hospice
Organization
St. Elizabeth Medical Center
110 S. Ninth Avenue
Yakima WA 98902
(509) 575-5163

Wyoming Hospice
Organization
Hospice of Sweetwater Co.
425 Centennial
Rock Springs WY 92935
(307) 362-1900

Visiting Nurses Association

(800-426-2547)
3801 East Florida, Suite 806
Denver CO 80210

The Visiting Nurses Association has four hundred and twenty offices nation wide. It is suggested you call the above toll-free number and discuss with them your location and potential needs. They will be able to direct you to the nearest available services offered by VNA. If there is no VNA office in your immediate vicinity, the home office will be able to advise you of other alternatives in your area.

National Cancer Institute

Office of Cancer Communications
Bethesda MD 20205
800-638-6694

The National Cancer Institute has offices in most of the fifty states with telephone services that offer information to the public and to health professionals. Information includes educational materials about cancer, information on the disease process, its treatment and emotional aspects and referral to appropriate treatment centers and local support and service organizations.

Dialing 1-800-4CANCER (1-800-422-6237) automatically routes your call to the local offices of the National Cancer Institute. If there is not a local office, your call is automatically routed to the national offices where they will be able to assist you in locating local services.

In Alaska, call 1-800-638-6070. In Hawaii, on Oahu, call 524-1234. Other islands, please call collect.

National Offices of Service Organizations

The following organizations are listed in the booklet *Taking Time*, published by the National Institutes of Health in the U.S. Department of Health and Human Services. You are encouraged to request a copy of this booklet from your nearest Cancer Institute Office by calling 1-800-4CANCER.

Cancer Care, Inc.
1180 Avenue of the Americas
New York NY 10036
212-302-2400

This is a service of the National Cancer Foundation and helps patients and families cope with the emotional, psychological and financial consequences of cancer at all stages of the illness. Services include home visits by trained volunteers, individual, family and group counseling, information referrals and assistance for nonmedical expenses.

Candlelighters Childhood Foundation, Inc.
Suite 1011
2025 I Street, N.W.
Washington DC 20006
202-659-5136

This is an international organization of parents whose children have or have had cancer. The foundation provides guidance, emotional support and referral services through self help and support groups. In addition to adolescent support groups and a youth newsletter, logistical support such as crisis intervention, babysitting and transportation is available. Some groups provide financial assistance.

CHUMS (Cancer Hopefuls United for Mutual Support)
3310 Rochambeau Avenue
Bronx NY 10467
212-655-7566

CHUMS is an organization of cancer survivors who offer emotional support to cancer patients and their families through self-help, crisis intervention, information, referrals and peer support.

Corporate Angel Network
Westchester County Airport, Building 1
White Plains NY 10604
914-328-1313

This organization assists cancer patients receiving special treatment in NCI-approved treatment centers by arranging for ambulatory patients and one attendant or family member to fly free on corporate aircraft when seats are available.

Leukemia Society of America, Inc.
733 Third Avenue
New York NY 10017
212-573-8484

Financial assistance, transportation and consultation services for referrals to other means of local support.

Make-a-Wish Foundation of America
4601 North 16th Street, Suite 205
Phoenix AZ 85016
602-234-0960

This organization works with families of terminally ill children up to the age of eighteen to cover expenses and arrange details necessary for granting a child's "special wish" to provide encouragement, respite from the current situation and special memories.

Make Today Count
P.O. Box 222
Osage Beach MO 65065
314-348-1619

Emotional self-help to assist patient and family to live each day as fully and completely as possible.

TOUCH
513 Tinsley Harrison Tower
University Station
Birmingham AL 35294
205-934-3814

Support groups assist cancer patients and their families in forming realistic, positive attitudes toward cancer and its treatment. Counselors guide support groups and assist in continuing education on treatment methods.

United Cancer Council, Inc.
650 East Carmel Drive, Suite 340
Carmel IN 46032
317-844-6627

A federation of voluntary cancer agencies funded through the United Way of Giving in most communities. Services include nursing, homemaking, housekeeping, medications, prostheses and rehabilitation.

United Ostomy Association, Inc.
2001 West Beverly Boulevard
Los Angeles CA 90057
213-413-5510

This group offers emotional support from others with common problems, mutual aid and education to those who have had colostomy, ileostomy or urostomy surgery.

We Can Do!
P.O. Box 723
Arcadia CA 91006
818-357-7517

This support program addresses the long-term psychological and educational needs of patients and their families, using groups, educational programs, referrals to local resources and classes for spouses of cancer patients.

Appendix F
Power
of Attorney

Know All Men By These Presents:

That _____has made, constituted and appointed, and by these presents does make, constitute and appoint _____ lawful attorney for _____ and in _____'s name, place and stead herewith giving and granting unto _____'s said attorney full power and authority to do and perform all and every act and thing whatsoever requisite and necessary to be done as fully, to all intents and purposes as _____ might or could do if personally present, with full power of substitution and revocation, hereby ratifying and confirming all that _____'s said attorney or his/her substitute shall lawfully do or cause to be done by virtue hereof.

In Witness Whereof, I have set my hand and seal this the_____day of_____,in the year 19_____.

Sealed and delivered in the presence of

_____   _____

_____   _____

State of

County of

Be It Known, That on the_____day of_____, 19____ before me,_____a_____in and for the State of Florida duly commissioned and sworn, dwelling in the_____personally came and appeared _____to me personally known, and known to me to be the same person described in and who executed the within power of attorney and who acknowledged the within power of attorney to be his/her act and deed.

In Testimony Whereof, I have hereunto subscribed my name and affixed my seal of office the day and year last above written.

Appendix G
Last Will and Testament

KNOW ALL MEN BY THESE PRESENTS: That I, of the City/Town of_____, and State of_____, being of sound and disposing mind and memory, do make, publish and declare the following to be my LAST WILL AND TESTAMENT, hereby revoking all Wills by me at any time heretofore made.

First: I direct my Executrix, hereinafter named, to pay all my funeral expenses, administration expenses of my estate, including any required inheritance and succession taxes, state or federal, which may be occasioned by the passage of or succession to any interest in my estate under the terms of either this instrument or a separate inter vivos trust instrument, and all my just debts, excepting mortgage notes secured by mortgages upon real estate.

Second: With the exception of the items listed in Section Three, I hereby give, devise and bequeath all the rest, residue and remainder of my estate, both real and personal, of whatsoever kind or character, and wheresoever situated to my husband/wife.

Third:

Fourth: In the event I am preceded in death by my Executor and Beneficiary_____, the following instructions regarding my estate are to be carried out by the Contingency Executrix,

Fifth: I hereby appoint_____, my wife/husband, as Executor of this my LAST WILL AND TESTAMENT. If he/she does not survive me, then I appoint as Executrix. I direct that no Executor/Executrix serving hereunder shall be required to post bond.

In Witness Whereof, I have hereunto set my hand and seal at this_____day of_____, 19____.

(signed)_____

Signed, sealed, published and declared to be his LAST WILL AND TESTAMENT by the within named testator in the presence of us, who in his presence and at his request, and in the presence of each other, have hereunto subscribed our names as witnesses:

(1)_____ of

_____
     City   State

(2)_____ of

_____
     City   State

(3)_____ of

_____
     City   State

AFFIDAVIT

State of_____

County of_____

Personally appeared

(1)_____

(2)_____ and

(3)_____

who being duly sworn, depose and say that they attested the said Will and they subscribed the same at the request and in the presence of the said Testator and in the presence of each other, and the said Testator signed said Will in their presence and acknowledged that he had signed said Will and declared the same to be his LAST WILL AND TESTAMENT, and deponents further state that at the time of the execution of said Will the said Testator appeared to be of lawful age and sound mind and memory and there was no evidence of undue influence. The deponents make this affidavit at the request of the Testator.

(1)_____

(2)_____

(3)_____

Subscribed and sworn to before me this_____day of _____,19_____.

(Notary Seal)

_____

Notary Public

Appendix H
Death with Dignity Direction

TO: My family, my physician, my lawyer, my clergyman;
TO: Any medical facility in whose care I happen to be;
TO: Any individual who may become responsible for my health, welfare, or affairs

Death is as much a reality as birth, growth, maturity and old age. It is the one certainty of life. If the time comes when I, _____, can no longer take part in decisions for my own future, let this statement stand as an expression of my wishes, while I am still capable of expressing my wishes.

I,_____, being of sound mind, willfully, and voluntarily make known my desire that my life shall not be artificially prolonged under the circumstances set forth below, and do hereby declare that:

(a) If at any time I should have an incurable injury, disease or illness certified to be a terminal condition by two physicians, and where the application of life-sustaining procedures would serve only to artificially prolong the moment of my death, and where my physician determines that my death is imminent whether or not life sustaining procedures are utilized, I direct that such procedures be withheld or withdrawn, and that I be permitted to die naturally;

(b) In the absence of my ability to give directions regarding the use of such life-sustaining procedures, it is my intention that this directive shall be honored by my family and physician(s) as the final expression of my legal right to refuse medical or surgical treatment and I accept the consequences from such refusal;

(c) If I have been diagnosed as pregnant, and that diagnosis is known to my physician, this directive shall have no force or effect during the course of my pregnancy;

(d) I understand the full import of this directive and I am emotionally and mentally competent to make this directive.

This directive is made after careful consideration. I hope you who care for me will feel morally bound to follow its mandate. I recognize that this appears to place a heavy responsibility upon you, but it is with the intention of relieving you of such responsibility and of placing it upon myself in accordance with my strong convictions, that this directive is made.

IN WITNESS WHEREOF, I,_____,
have set my hand this_____day of_____, 19____

_____(Name)
_____(Address)
_____(Address)

The declarer has been personally known to me and I believe him/her to be of sound mind. I am not related to the declarer, nor will I gain by his/her death. I am not associated with any person or organization who provides health care services to the declarer..

DATED THIS_____day of_____, 19___.

WITNESS_____

WITNESS_____

THIS DIRECTIVE IS INTENDED TO COMPLY WITH RCW 70.122

O R D E R   F O R M

☐ **PLEASE SEND ME A FREE CATALOG**

Name_____

Address_____

City_____State_____Zip_____

Quantity	Book Title and Author	Price	Total
	The Other Side of the Closet: The Coming-Out Crisis for Straight Spouses by Amity Pierce Buxton, Ph.D.	$ 14.95	
	When Someone You Love Has Cancer by Dana Rae Pomeroy	9.95	
	When Women Choose to be Single by Rita Robinson	9.95	
	When Your Parents Need You: A Caregiver's Guide by Rita Robinson	9.95	
	Survivors of Suicide by Rita Robinson	9.95	
	Good People: The Whole Self Integration Guide by Ruth Cherry, Ph.D.	12.95	
	Master Meditations: A Spiritual Daybook by Dr. Donald Curtis	12.95	
	The Book of Rituals: Personal and Planetary Transformation by Rev. Carol Parrish-Harra	14.95	
	The New Age Handbook on Death and Dying by Rev. Carol Parrish-Harra	8.95	
	The Law of Mind in Action by Dr. Fenwicke Lindsay Holmes	10.95	
	Axioms for Survivors: A Caregivers Guide by Lon Nungesser, M.A.	6.95	
	Being Human in the Face of Death edited by Deborah Roth, MSC & Emily LeVier, MSC	9.95	
	Stepping Stones to Grief Recovery edited by Deborah Roth, MSC	8.95	
	AIDS: A Self-Care Manual (Third Edition) by AIDS Project Los Angeles	14.95	
	When Someone You Love Has AIDS by BettyClare Moffatt, MA	8.95	
	Gifts for the Living: Conversations with Caregivers on Death and Dying by BettyClare Moffatt, MA	9.95	

Please send check or money order to:	SUBTOTAL
IBS Press, Inc. 744 Pier Avenue Santa Monica, CA 90405 (213)450-6485 (213)314-8268 (FAX)	SALES TAX 6.5% (California Only)
	SHIPPING/HANDLING ($2.00 per book)
	TOTAL DUE

ORDERS   1-800-234-6485
VISA & MASTERCARD ACCEPTED
Weekdays, 9:00 am - 5:00 pm PST

IBS PRESS, Inc
744 Pier Avenue
Santa Monica, CA 90405